Oxford Case Histories in Sleep Medicine

Oxford Case Histories
Series Editors
Sarah Pendlebury and Peter Rothwell

Oxford Case Histories in Neurosurgery (Harutomo Hasegawa, Matthew Crocker, and Pawan Singh Minhas)

Oxford Case Histories in TIA and Stroke (Sarah T. Pendlebury, Ursula G. Schulz, Aneil Malhotra, and Peter M. Rothwell)

Oxford Case Histories in Rheumatology (Joel David, Anne Miller, Anushka Soni, and Lyn Williamson)

Oxford Case Histories in Cardiology (Rajkumar Rajendram, Javed Ehtisham, and Colin Forfar)

Oxford Case Histories in Respiratory Medicine (John Stradling, Andrew Stanton, Najib M. Rahman, Annabel H. Nickol, and Helen E. Davies)

Oxford Case Histories in Gastroenterology and Hepatology (Alissa J. Walsh, Otto C. Buchel, Jane Collier, and Simon P. L. Travis)

Neurological Case Histories (Sarah T. Pendlebury, Philip Anslow, and Peter M. Rothwell)

Oxford Case Histories in Sleep Medicine

Himender Makker

Consultant Physician in Respiratory Medicine,
North Middlesex University and University College
London (UCL) Hospital, London, UK

Matthew Walker

Professor of Neurology, UCL Institute of Neurology,
Queen Square, London, UK

Hugh Selsick

Psychiatrist, Camden and Islington NHS Trust London
and the Royal London Hospital for Integrated Medicine,
London, UK

Bhik Kotecha

Consultant ENT Surgeon and Lead Clinician for Snoring
and Sleep Service, The Royal National Throat Nose
and Ear Hospital, UCL, London, and Barking, Havering
and Redbridge University Hospital, London, UK

Ama Johal

Senior Clinical Lecturer/Hon. Consultant Orthodontist
Academic and Clinical Lead Orthodontics Institute
of Dentistry Bart's, and The London School of Medicine
and Dentistry, Queen Mary College, London, UK

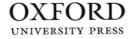

OXFORD
UNIVERSITY PRESS

OXFORD
UNIVERSITY PRESS

Great Clarendon Street, Oxford, OX2 6DP,
United Kingdom

Oxford University Press is a department of the University of Oxford.
It furthers the University's objective of excellence in research, scholarship,
and education by publishing worldwide. Oxford is a registered trade mark of
Oxford University Press in the UK and in certain other countries

First Edition published in 2015
Impression: 1

Published in the United States of America by Oxford University Press
198 Madison Avenue, New York, NY 10016, United States of America

British Library Cataloguing in Publication Data
Data available

Library of Congress Control Number: 2014955874

ISBN 978–0–19–968395–6

Printed in Great Britain by
Clays Ltd, St Ives plc

Preface

Our interest in sleep disorders is relatively new in the history of medicine. The ability to measure physiological events during sleep has led to the recognition of previously unknown sleep disorders. Basic understanding of structure and function of normal sleep has made us realise the importance of sleep on quality of life, health, and survival. A better understanding of sleep disorders has helped us to develop new treatments.

Despite immense advances in the understanding and management of sleep disorders over the last 50 years, many sleep disorders remain under-diagnosed and under-treated. Opportunities for teaching and training in sleep medicine remain limited. Available learning resources for sleep medicine are primarily aimed at sleep specialists, leaving a gap for non-sleep specialists.

This book provides a case-based illustrative approach to the understanding and management of common and important sleep disorders—snoring, sleep disordered breathing, insomnia, circadian-rhythm disorders, and primary neurological sleep disorders. Case histories have been written by sleep medicine experts with clinical experience of providing a multi-disciplinary sleep service. Case examples have been selected direct from sleep clinics and focus on the recognition of presenting features of sleep disorders and their clinical importance. Each case report provides a detailed clinical description followed by a clear explanation of the salient points. The text is supported by photographs, diagrams, and line drawings, and concludes with a list of key learning points. An attempt has been made to write the cases in an easy-flowing prose to simulate the experience of seeing and discussing a real-life patient in a clinic. The book will be of interest to all clinicians who wish to improve their understanding and knowledge of sleep disorders.

I wish to thank my following colleagues for their contribution to Obstructive sleep apnoea and ENT sections of the book: Dr Fionnuala Crummy, Consultant Respiratory Physician, University College London Hospital, London and Mr Rob Nash, Specialist ENT Registrar, Royal National Throat, Nose and Ear Hospital, London.

I also wish to thank Peter Stevenson and Lauren Dunn at the Oxford University Press for their constant support and encouragement, my co-authors for providing excellent case histories, and my secretary, Donna Basire, for checking the manuscript tirelessly.

Himender Makker

Contents

List of abbreviations

ABG	arterial blood gases	EEG	Electroencephalogram
ACE	angiotensin converting enzyme	EMG	electromyogram
AHI	apnoea hypopnea index	ENT	ear, nose and throat
AHRF	acute hypercapnic respiratory failure	EOG	electroculogram
ANP	atrial natriuretic peptide	EPAP	Expiratory Positive Airway Pressure
ASPS	advanced sleep phase syndrome	ESS	Epworth Sleepiness Scale
ASV	adaptive servo-ventilation	FEV1	Forced Expiratory Volume in first second
BiPAP	bi-level positive airway pressure	FLEP	frontal lobe epilepsy and parasomnias scale
BMI	body mass index	FRC	functional residual capacity
BPD	bilio-pancreatic diversion	FSHD	fascioscapulohumeral dystrophy
BPH	benign prostatic hypertrophy	FVC	forced vital capacity
CBT	Cognitive Behavioural Therapy	GCS	Glasgow Coma Scale
CBT-I	cognitive behavioural therapy for insomnia	GH	growth hormone
CNS	central nervous system	GORD	gastro-oesophageal reflux disease
COPD	chronic obstructive pulmonary disease	HDU	High Dependency Unit
CPAP	continuous positive airway pressure	HLA	human leukocyte antigen
		ICD	Implantable Cardioverter Defibrillator
CRP	C-reactive protein	IGF	insulin-like growth factor
CRT	cardiac resynchronization therapy	IPAP	Inspiratory Positive Airway Pressure
CRT-D	Cardiac Resynchronization Therapy Device	ITU	intensive therapy unit
CSA	central sleep apnoea	LAUP	laser assisted uvulopalatoplasty
CSF	cerebrospinal fluid	LPR	laryngo-pharyngo reflux
CSR	Cheyne–Stokes respiration	MAD	mandibular advancement device
DaT	Dopamine transporter		
DAT	dopamine transporters	MAS	mandibular advancement splint
DLMO	dim light melatonin onset		
DSPS	delayed sleep phase syndrome	MDSA	medical dental sleep appliance
DVLA	Driver Vehicle Licensing Agency	MEFV	maximum expiratory flow volume
ECG	electrocardiogram	MIFV	maximum inspiratory flow volume
EDS	excessive daytime sleepiness		

MRD	mandibular repositioning devices
MRI	magnetic resonance imaging
MSLT	multiple sleep latency time
MWT	maintenance of wakefulness test
NIV	non-invasive ventilation
NREM	Non-rapid eye movement
OSAS	obstructive sleep apnoea syndrome
ODI	Oxygen Desaturation Index
OHS	obesity hypoventilation syndrome
OSA	obstructive sleep apnoea
OSAHS	obstructive sleep apnoea hypopnoea syndrome
PCA	patient controlled analgesia
PLMS	periodic limb movement syndrome
PSG	Polysomnography
PSV	Public Service Vehicle
RAST	radioallergosorbent test
RBD	REM sleep behavioural disorder
RDI	Respiratory Distress Index
REM	rapid eye movement
RERA	respiratory effort related arousal
RHT	retinohypothalamic tract
RLS	restless legs syndrome
RR	distance between R, two consecutive waves on ECG (heart rate)
RTA	road traffic accident
RYGB	Roux en Y gastric bypass
SAD	seasonal affective disorder
SCN	Supra Chiasmatic Nucleus
SDB	Sleep Disordered Breathing
SE	sleep efficiency
SOL	sleep onset latency
SPECT	single-photon emission computerized tomography
SSRI	selective serotonin reuptake inhibitor
SWD	shift work disorder
TIB	time in bed
TMJ	temporomandibular joints
TST	total sleep time
UARS	upper airway resistance syndrome
UPPP	uvulopalatopharyngoplasty
VLPA	ventro-lateral pre-optic area
WASO	wakefulness after sleep onset

Normal ranges

Hb	13–18g/dL (men)
	11.5–16g/dL (women)
MCV	76–96fL
WCC	$4–11 \times 10^9$/L
Plt	$150–400 \times 10^9$/L
Na	135–145mmol/L
K	3.5–5mmol/L
Urea	2.5–6.7mmol/L
Cr	70–150µmol/L
Ca	2.12–2.65mmol/L
CK	25–195IU/L
CRP	<10mg/L
Glc (fasting)	3.5–5.5mmol/L
Bili	3–17µmol/L
AST	3–35IU/L
Alk phosp	30–300IU/L
GGT	11–51IU/L (men), 7–33IU/L (women)

Blood gases

PH	7.35–7.45
PaO2	>10.6kPa
PaCO2	4.7–6kPa
Bicarbonate	24–30mmol/L

CSF

Protein	0.15–0.45g/L
glc	2.8–4.2mmol/L
WCC	<5 lymphocytes/mm^3
Opening pressure	7–18cm H_2O

Section 1

Snoring and sleep-disordered breathing

Case 1
Snoring and witnessed apnoea in a 70-year-old thin man

A 70-year-old Chinese man was referred to the sleep clinic because his friends were worried about his loud snoring and the fact that he stopped breathing during sleep when he stayed with them for a week after his wife's death. He slept alone and well, and had no breathing difficulties during sleep. He woke up fresh from his sleep and did not experience any daytime sleepiness or tiredness. He reported no reduction in his concentration or impairment of his memory. He did not have any headaches or any recent change in weight. He had a blocked nose and woke up with a dry throat in the morning. He had a myocardial infarction in the past for which he had an angioplasty. His hyperlipidaemia and hypertension were controlled on treatment. There was no family history of sleep apnoea or snoring. He was a retired caterer and non-smoker, and did not drink alcohol. He was of normal body weight with a body mass index (BMI) of 19.9 and his neck size was 35 centimetres. However, his oral cavity was narrow—Mallampati score 3 out of 4. His blood pressure was 140/95 mmHg, his resting oxygen saturations were 97% on air, and, on the Epworth Sleepiness Scale (ESS), he scored 0 out of 24.

A multichannel home sleep study confirmed the diagnosis of obstructive sleep apnoea (OSA). His apnoea hypopnea index (AHI) was 26 with an oxygen desaturation dip rate of 21.7, and mean oxygen saturations were normal at 97%. A total of 117 snoring episodes were recorded and he snored for a total of 25 minutes. He slept in the supine position during most of the night. His AHI consisted of 62% of obstructive apnoeas and 37% hypopnoeas. The longest apnoea was of 64 seconds duration with a mean duration of apnoea at 32 seconds (Figures 1.1–1.4).

Sleep Summary

Apnea/Hypopnea		
Index Time:	446.9 minutes	
Apnea + Hypopnea (A+H):	194	26.0/h
Supine A+H:	193	26.5/h
Non-Supine A+H:	1	6.1/h
Position		
Supine Time:	437.2 minutes	97.8 %
Non-Supine Time:	9.8 minutes	2.2 %
Upright Time:	2.7 minutes	0.6 %
Movement Time:	18.3 minutes	4.1 %
Oxygen Saturation		
Average Oxygen Saturation:	97.0 %	
Oxygen Desaturation Events (OD):	162	21.7/h
Snoring		
Snore Time:	25.0 minutes	5.6 %
Number of Snoring Episodes:	117	

Fig. 1.1 Sleep study summary data confirming moderately severe OSA (AHI 26) associated with oxygen desaturations (SaO$_2$ 4% dip rate 21.7) and snoring.

He was fitted with a nasal continuous positive airway pressure (CPAP) mask and treated with an auto-CPAP machine. A repeat sleep study on CPAP showed that his sleep apnoea had completely subsided and AHI was 0.1. His mean oxygen saturations were normal at 96.7% and the oxygen desaturation dip rate was 0.1. The snoring was completely

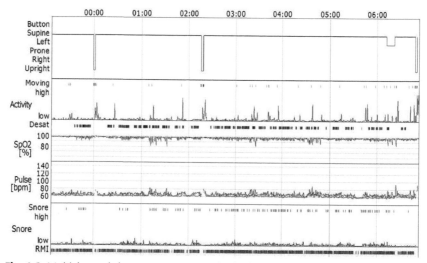

Fig. 1.2 Multichannel sleep measurements: body sleep position, activity, SaO$_2$, pulse, and snoring monitoring in an OSA patient.

Summary Graph

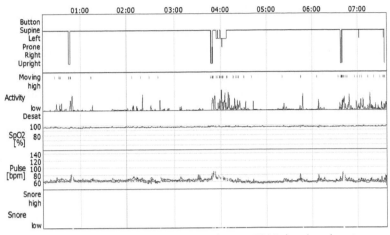

Fig. 1.3 Sleep study summary data in an OSA patient on CPAP showing almost complete elimination of apnoeas, oxygen desaturations, and snoring.

eliminated on CPAP (Figures 1.3 and 1.4). The CPAP pressure setting showed that the median CPAP pressure required was 7.1 cm of water. A CPAP compliance check showed that he used his CPAP for 15 out of 17 days with a median daily use of 3.28 hours. He reported an improvement in his sleep quality.

Sleep Summary

Apnea/Hypopnea		
Index Time:	414.7 minutes	
Apnea + Hypopnea (A+H):	1	0.1 / h
Supine A+H:	1	0.1 / h
Non-Supine A+H:	0	0.0 / h
Position		
Supine Time:	408.1 minutes	98.4 %
Non-Supine Time:	6.6 minutes	1.6 %
Upright Time:	3.2 minutes	0.8 %
Movement Time:	30.1 minutes	7.3 %
Oxygen Saturation		
Average Oxygen Saturation:	96.7 %	
Oxygen Desaturation Events (OD):	1	0.1 / h
Snoring		
Snore Time:	- minutes	- %
Number of Snoring Episodes:	-	

Fig. 1.4 Multichannel sleep measurements in patients with OSA on CPAP: body sleep position, activity, SaO$_2$, pulse, and snoring in an OSA patient.

However, despite good initial compliance, he returned the CPAP machine a year later because of symptoms of nasal itching, dryness of throat and bringing up blood from his throat in the morning. ENT examination and CT scan of his head and neck showed no cause of the nasal symptoms and apparent epistaxis/haemoptysis. He was provided with a custom-made mono-block mandibular advancement splint. He used his splint every night, throughout the night, with no side effects and reported an improvement in his dryness of throat and no further bringing up of blood from the back of the throat. A sleep study with a mandibular advancement splint in situ showed no sleep apnoea.

Questions

1 How common is OSA?

2 What are the main risk factors for OSA?

3 What are the main presenting features of OSA?

4 What are good clinical predictors of OSA?

5 How do you confirm the diagnosis of OSA?

6 Is there a correlation between symptoms of OSA and the severity measured on a sleep study?

narrow nose and use devices such as nasal dilator strips or a nasal valve, which rarely work. Snoring, like sleep apnoea, comes from the back of the throat, the back of the tongue and the soft palate. Many snorers snore louder when they sleep on their back due to the tongue and palate falling back, and treatment is based on preventing snorers sleeping on their back—positional treatments such as fixing a tennis ball to the back of pyjamas have been attempted, but are rarely successful in the long term. They are unable to comply with these treatments because of the discomfort and inconvenience associated with sleeping in one particular position. Surgical treatment for snoring such as laser assisted uvulopalatoplasty (LAUP), which is thought to work by stiffening the soft palate, may work for some patients in the short term. However, a mandibular advancement splint (dental splint, mouth guard) which works by keeping the lower jaw forward during sleep (the lower jaw often drops back during sleep due to muscle relaxation and narrows the upper airway further) is an effective and non-invasive treatment. Finally, lifestyle changes—weight loss, improved fitness and avoidance of alcohol before sleep—can significantly improve snoring.

Witnessed apnoea: this is a common presenting feature of OSA. The episodes of witnessed apnoea can be fairly prolonged, lasting up to a minute, and can worry their bed partner who often shake/wake them to start breathing. Snorers with a history of witnessed apnoeas are much more likely to have OSA than a simple snorer. However, the apnoeas may not be witnessed if the patient sleeps alone or if their partner fails to notice. A few patients report disturbed sleep due to choking or gasping for breath.

EDS: this is a common symptom among the general population— surveys have found that 50% of people have some degree of daytime sleepiness. True daytime sleepiness should be distinguished from fatigue, tiredness, or lethargy. EDS can be due to either lack of sleep (duration–quantity) or poor quality sleep. OSA patients often report sleeping for long hours, but still wake up unrefreshed and feel sleepy during the daytime due to recurrent arousals during sleep affecting their quality of sleep (reduced slow wave and REM sleep). The ESS questionnaire is one of the most commonly used in the assessment of EDS. EDS is a common presentation of OSA, but it can be due to a variety of other causes.

Patients with a combination of symptoms—snoring associated with witnessed apnoeas and daytime sleepiness—are much more likely to have OSA than patients with only one of these symptoms.

4. What are good clinical predictors of OSA?

OSA is due to the narrowing and increased collapsibility of the upper airway. Obesity (BMI >30) and an increase in neck size (collar >17) are easily visible risk factors for OSA. Subtle craniofacial skeletal abnormalities may be difficult to recognize on inspection—but a small and receded jaw (retrognathia and micrognathia) is an obvious risk factor for OSA. It reduces the space for the tongue, pushing it back and narrowing the upper airways. Simple visual inspection of the oral cavity and an assessment of the oral cavity size using a Mallampati score is a good tool for assessing the risk of OSA—patients with a grade 3 or 4 size oral cavity are at a high risk of OSA. Imaging techniques such as CT and MRI scans can clearly demonstrate narrow upper airways, but their use should be restricted for complex patients with a suspected anatomical obstructing lesion of the upper airway.

In summary, obese people with a big neck or people of normal body weight with a small jaw and narrow oral cavity presenting with loud disruptive snoring associated with witnessed apnoeas and EDS should be suspected to have sleep apnoea and referred for a sleep study.

Different sleep questionnaires use combination of the clinical features described here to predict or determine the risk of OSA.

5. How do you confirm the diagnosis of OSA?

Clinical features are useful to determine the increased risk of OSA in patients, but none is sensitive enough to confirm nor specific enough to rule out the diagnosis of OSA. A sleep study is required to confirm the diagnosis. A polysomnography (PSG) sleep study was thought to be gold standard. However, it is complex and expensive, and is not

Questions

1 Does nasal obstruction cause or contribute to snoring and OSA?

2 What is the natural history of a snorer?

3 Is there an effect of gender on OSA?

4 What are the possible reasons for gender differences in the prevalence and severity of OSA?

5 Do sex hormones contribute to the difference in OSA between the two genders?

Answers

1. Does nasal obstruction cause or contribute to snoring and OSA?

Snoring and obstructive sleep apnoea are mainly caused by obstruction of the upper airway at the level of the soft palate and tongue base and is rarely due to obstruction to the nose. Most devices aimed at improving nasal flow, such as nasal dilator devices for treatment of snoring, are ineffective. However, nasal obstruction with associated symptoms may cause disturbed sleep and dry throat due to mouth breathing. Similarly, patients with nasal obstruction find difficulty in using a nasal CPAP mask.

2. What is the natural history of a snorer?

Loud snoring is often a warning sign for OSA. An increase in body weight and reduced level of fitness in a snorer can cause obstructive sleep apnoea. Initially, a snorer has intermittent apnoeas usually precipitated by factors such as excessive alcohol consumption, supine body position, or deep sleep. However, at the later stages, with progressive weight gain they may obstruct every night and during all body positions and sleep stages.

3. Is there an effect of gender on OSA?

Middle-aged men are more likely to be suspected of having OSA and referred to a sleep clinic than women. Therefore, in the sleep clinic population, more men have OSA than women—a ratio as high as 10:1. This can give an erroneous impression that OSA is mainly a disease of middle-aged obese men. However, population studies have shown that gender difference in the prevalence of OSA is much lower at a ratio of 2:1. It is likely that a lower index of suspicion of OSA and referral to a sleep clinic accounts for a higher gender difference in the clinic population. It is also possible that there are gender differences in the perception and reporting of OSA symptoms— women may under-report their snoring because of embarrassment. Their perception of daytime sleepiness is different and their threshold for reporting sleepiness can be higher than men. Surveys have shown that self-reported sleepiness on an ESS score is often lower in women than men. Moreover, women tend to notice their partner/husbands snoring and witness apnoeas more often than men, and prompt them to seek help. Finally, men presenting with symptoms of OSA to the GP are more likely to be referred to a sleep clinic than women due to a difference in the description of the symptoms by two genders. Women often report daytime sleepiness and sleep disturbance as fatigue and the inability to sleep (insomnia). This is more likely to be labelled due to depression than sleep apnoea. Nevertheless, despite lower differences in the prevalence of OSA between men and women, severe and symptomatic OSA is much more common in men than women.

4. What are the possible reasons for gender differences in the prevalence and severity of OSA?

It is a common observation that obese women are bigger around the lower part of the body (gynoid distribution) than men who put on weight in the upper part of the body. Obese women tend to maintain their neck size, while obese men have big necks. Neck obesity (collar size >17) causes narrowing of the upper airway and is a much better predictor of OSA than BMI. Imaging studies have also shown that men have longer and more collapsible airways than women. Similarly, visceral obesity is a better predictor of OSA than BMI—this is thought to be related to visceral fat inflammatory cytokines which affect the central ventilatory control of breathing. Furthermore, for the same degrees of obesity men are more likely to have lower lung volumes than women. The combination of differences in obesity causes more prolonged apnoeas and hypoxia for the same degree of obstruction in men as women.

5. Do sex hormones contribute to the difference in OSA between the two genders?

Gender difference in prevalence of OSA is much more marked between premenopausal women and men, and relatively small between postmenopausal women and men. Furthermore, postmenopausal women on HRT have lower prevalence of OSA. The lower prevalence of OSA in premenopausal woman and postmenopausal women on HRT is thought to be due to the protective effect of oestrogen and progesterone on the risk of OSA. Oestrogen promotes gynoid lower-body fat distribution in premenopausal women and postmenopausal woman on HRT, and progesterone has a respiratory stimulant effect.

Learning points

Snoring and OSA are caused by the narrowing of the upper airway at the pharynx. Nasal obstruction may worsen snoring and OSA, but is rarely a cause in itself.

Snoring may be a warning sign of OSA. This can progress to OSA with weight gain.

Lower prevalence of OSA in obese premenopausal woman than men is due to differences in fat distribution of lower body versus upper body.

Further reading

Lin CM, Davidson TM, Ancoli-Israel S. Gender differences in obstructive sleep apnea and treatment implications. Sleep Med Rev 2008 Dec;12(6):481–96.

Parker RJ, Hardinge M, Jeffries C. Snoring. BMJ 2005 Nov;331(7524):1063. Review.

Case 3
Severe OSA in an overweight Chinese man—craniofacial features

Mr KK, a 35-year-old Chinese man, was diagnosed to have severe OSA in Hong Kong. His sleep study showed a Respiratory Distress Index (RDI) of 73.7. The longest duration of apnoea was 97 seconds and the lowest SaO_2 was 53%. He was treated with CPAP at a fixed pressure of 12 cm of water. He lived in the UK and was referred to a sleep clinic for follow-up. He had micrognathia and retrognathia, and a long, floppy uvula. He was overweight, weighing 80.8 kg for a height of 175.2 cm (BMI 26) and his collar size was 17 (43 cm). He reported an improvement in symptoms of OSA with CPAP, but had difficulty in tolerating CPAP because of high CPAP pressure.

His baseline sleep study off CPAP (three days) confirmed severe OSA with a SaO_2 dip rate of 74/hour and nocturnal hypoxia—the mean SaO_2 was 90.84% and the lowest SaO_2 65%, and Total Sleep Time $<SaO_2$ of 90% (TST <90) was 2.45 hours (48%). His CPAP pressure was reduced to 10 cm of water, with an improvement in CPAP tolerance. Repeat sleep study on CPAP showed a dip rate of 0.78/hour and a mean SaO_2 of 97.25%. He has been using CPAP for the last ten years.

Questions

1 What are the craniofacial features associated with OSA and how can you detect these features?

2 What is the contribution of craniofacial features to the prevalence of OSA in different ethnic populations?

3 What are the clinical implications of craniofacial abnormalities in OSA?

Table 3.1 Craniofacial features commonly associated with OSA

Skeletal	Soft tissues
Maxilla	Tongue
• Shorter maxillary length	• Enlarged
• Maxillary constriction	Soft palate
Mandible	• Enlarged
• Shorter corpus length	• Longer uvula
• Retropositioning	Parapharyngeal fat pads
• Steep mandibular plane	• Larger volume
• Smaller mandibular enclosure area	Lateral pharyngeal walls
Hyoid	• Greater pharyngeal wall width
• Inferiorly positioned	• Larger volume
Cranial base	Upper airway
• Narrow anterior base	• Smaller airway space
• Acute cranial base flexure	Anatomical balance
Face and head position	• Larger tongue for bony craniofacial enclosure size
• Longer anterior face height	
• Extended head position	

Source: Sutherland K, Lee RW, Cistulli PA. Obesity and craniofacial structure as risk factors for obstructive sleep apnoea: impact of ethnicity. Respirology. 2012 Feb;17(2):213–22. doi: 10.1111/j.1440–1843.2011.02082.x. Review. PubMed PMID: 21,992,683.

2. What is the contribution of craniofacial features to the prevalence of OSA in different ethnic populations?

Until recently, OSA was thought to be less common in the Chinese and Asian population because of a relatively low prevalence of obesity compared to the White Caucasian population. However, recent population studies have shown that the prevalence of OSA is as high in Chinese and Asian ethnic groups as in the White Caucasian population. Craniofacial features in Chinese people favour retro-positioning of the mandible as a main risk factor for OSA. A study found that Chinese Hong Kong patients with OSA had a smaller mandible, maxilla and cranial base than the white Canadian population.

3. What are the clinical implications of craniofacial abnormalities in OSA?

Obese White Caucasian people with a smaller mandible, maxilla and cranial base, and an inferiorly placed hypoid are more likely to develop OSA than obese patients without these abnormalities. Similarly, Asian people may develop OSA with a mild degree of obesity or without obesity compared to the White Caucasian patients because

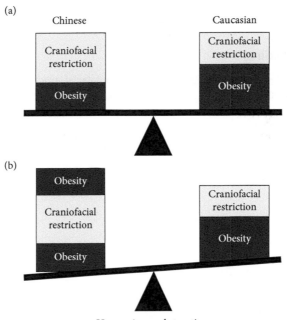

Upper airway obstruction

Fig. 3.3 Anatomical balance in OSA. The balance between the relative size of the craniofacial bony compartment and degree of obesity is an important determinant of upper airway obstruction. (a) Influence of ethnicity on anatomical balance. Degree of anatomical imbalance between Caucasian and Chinese OSA patients may be equivalent; however, the relative portions of obesity versus craniofacial bony restriction contributing to anatomic imbalance appear to be different between these ethnicities. (b) In this scenario, Chinese OSA patients with a restricted bony compartment may be more vulnerable to weight gain, as excess obesity will further exacerbate anatomical imbalance.

Source: Reproduced with permission from Sutherland, K, Lee, R. W. W., and Cistulli, P. A. (2012), Obesity and craniofacial structure as risk factors for obstructive sleep apnoea: Impact of ethnicity. Respirology, 17: 213–222. © 2011 The Authors. Respirology © 2011 Asian Pacific Society of Respirology.

of their craniofacial features (see Figure 3.3). Non-CPAP treatments, such as a mandibular advancement splint and surgical advancement of the mandible and maxilla, may have a more important role in OSA patients with craniofacial abnormalities.

Learning points

Not all obese patients have sleep apnoea and the absence of obesity does not exclude OSA.

Craniofacial features (often genetic/racial) can cause OSA and increase the severity of OSA due to obesity.

Further reading

Sutherland K, Lee RW, Cistulli PA. Obesity and craniofacial structure as risk factors for obstructive sleep apnoea: impact of ethnicity. Respirology 2012 Feb;17(2):213–22.

Case 4
Unable to throw a cricket ball and could not breathe at night

A 56-year-old man was referred by an ENT surgeon for the management of suspected OSA. He had fluctuating nasal obstruction due to mild nasal septum deviation towards the left, but was not keen on surgical correction. He snored heavily seven nights a week and also had episodes of witnessed apnoeas. He had disturbed sleep with frequent arousals. He woke up unrefreshed from his sleep with marked daytime sleepiness—mainly affecting him post-lunch. He was not obese, but had put on approximately one stone in weight over the preceding two years. He worked as a chartered accountant, did not smoke and drank alcohol on a social basis.

He was diagnosed to have fascioscapulohumeral dystrophy (FSHD) at the age of 18 years when he could not throw a cricket ball. His muscle weakness had progressed and mobility has deteriorated gradually over the last five years. He was unable to get about independently and was usually accompanied by his wife. He had starting using a walking stick and was considering using a mobility scooter. His father had muscular dystrophy and his daughter has genetically confirmed FSHD.

His BMI was 26.5 and his collar size was 41.5 cm. On oral cavity examination, his Mallampati score was normal at 2. His pulmonary function tests showed normal forced vital capacity (FVC) of 5.03 litres (103.7% of predicted) and FEV1 was normal at 4.02 (101% of predicted). His resting oxygen saturations were normal at 96%. His daytime sleepiness score—ESS—was high at 15 out of 24. Neurological review confirmed peri-clavicular thinning of muscles and shoulder girdle atrophy with mild scapular winging on the right side. He had mild weakness of the shoulder, elbow muscles and finger muscles, and bilateral foot drop with a high stepping gait. He did not have any retinal lens dysplasia and his blood pressure was normal at 123/84 mmHg. His routine blood test, full blood count, white cell count, ESR, urea and electrolytes, plasma glucose, serum lipids and thyroid function tests were all within normal limits. His chest X-ray was normal.

A sleep study confirmed severe OSA. His AHI was 47.9 with an oxygen desaturation dip rate of 39/hour and mean oxygen saturations during sleep of 94.7%. The apnoeas were mainly obstructive—the longest apnoea lasted for 87.7 seconds and the mean duration of apnoeas was 27 seconds. The total time spent below oxygen saturation of 90% was 2.8%, a total of 11 minutes. He was commenced on auto-CPAP and this completely corrected his sleep apnoea—the AHI normalized to 0.7. A CPAP compliance check showed that he used CPAP every night for a median duration of 7.3 hours. He noticed impressive improvement in his sleep quality which was refreshing and he was not sleepy during the daytime. He used to have early morning headaches, and these subsided. According to his wife, he had no further snoring or obstructive breathing.

Questions

1 What is the role of upper airways muscles in pathogenesis of OSA?

2 What are the common neuromuscular conditions that affect upper airway muscles?

3 How common is sleep apnoea in FSH muscular dystrophy?

4 Does upper airway muscle training, strengthening or stimulation have a role in the treatment of OSA?

Answers

1. What is the role of upper airways muscles in pathogenesis of OSA?

Upper airway (pharyngeal) muscles have an important role in maintaining upper airway patency, both during wakefulness and sleep, to allow unobstructed breathing. There are four groups of upper airway muscles—the tongue, palatal, hyoid and pharyngeal muscles. The coordinated action of these muscles maintains patency of the upper airway during breathing. Tongue muscle contraction, notably genioglossus, keeps the tongue forward (protrusion) with an increase in oropharynx size and stiffens the tongue to prevent upper airway collapsibility. Palatal muscles open or close nasal airways and promote nasal or mouth breathing. Hyoid muscle contraction enlarges the upper airway by bringing the hyoid forward and down. Pharyngeal constrictors mainly help with swallowing.

During wakefulness, the pharyngeal muscles are active and keep the upper airways open. However, during sleep or sedation (alcohol, sedatives and general anaesthesia), the muscle activity is depressed, resulting in upper airways narrowing and increases in resistance to airflow (see Figure 4.1). The upper airways are collapsible during sleep and prone to partial or complete obstruction. In people with a normal upper airway anatomy, upper airway collapse generates mechanoreceptor, hypercapnic and hypoxic stimuli to upper muscles during sleep to restore the patency of the upper airways and breathing. However, in patients with anatomically narrow upper airways, an increase in activity of the upper airway dilator muscles is not sufficient to overcome sleep-related upper airway obstruction. Upper airway muscles in patients with OSA are intrinsically normal—in fact, they work harder to keep the upper airways open. However, in patients with neuromuscular disorders causing muscle weakness, upper airways are vulnerable to collapse during sleep, even in the absence of any anatomical abnormality of the upper airways. In patients with upper airway muscle weakness due to disorders such as syringomyelia and motor neurone disease, other functions of the upper airway

(a)

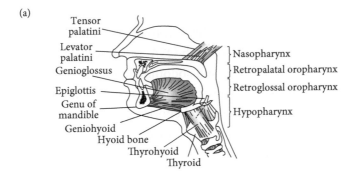

Tensor palatini
Levator palatini
Genioglossus
Epiglottis
Genu of mandible
Geniohyoid
Hyoid bone
Thyrohyoid
Thyroid

Nasopharynx
Retropalatal oropharynx
Retroglossal oropharynx
Hypopharynx

(b)

cartilage

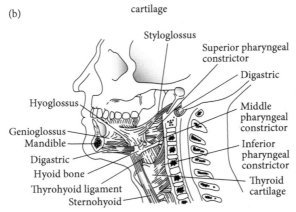

Styloglossus
Superior pharyngeal constrictor
Digastric
Hyoglossus
Genioglossus
Mandible
Digastric
Hyoid bone
Thyrohyoid ligament
Sternohyoid
Middle pharyngeal constrictor
Inferior pharyngeal constrictor
Thyroid cartilage

Fig. 4.1 Showing pharyngeal muscles involved in controlling upper airway patency during sleep and wakefulness.
Source: Reproduced with permission from Edwards BA, White DP. Control of the pharyngeal musculature during wakefulness and sleep: implications in normal controls and sleep apnea. Head Neck. 2011Oct;33 Suppl 1:S37-45. © 2011 Wiley Periodicals, Inc.

muscles, such as swallowing and speech, are also affected. Episodes of choking on swallowing, weakness of voice and choking/difficulty during sleep should prompt investigation for OSA.

2. What are the common neuromuscular conditions that affect upper airway muscles?

The upper airway muscles can be affected by various neuromuscular disorders, and weakness of the upper airway muscles not only impairs swallowing and speech, but increases their collapsibility, particularly during sleep, and causes OSA. Neuromuscular diseases causing weakness of bulbar muscles, such as amyotrophic lateral sclerosis, Duchene muscular dystrophy, myotonic dystrophy and myasthenia gravis, are often associated with OSA. Most sleep studies rely on the measurement of thoracic and abdominal movements during apnoea to differentiate between obstructive and central apnoea—cessation of airflow with thoracoabdominal effort/movement is characterized as obstructive apnoea and no movement as central apnoea. This may lead to misclassification of obstructive as central apnoea (pseudo-central apnoea). Sleep studies using oesophageal pressure monitoring can help to differentiate central from obstructive apnoea accurately.

3. How common is sleep apnoea in FSH muscular dystrophy?

FSH muscular dystrophy is an autosomal dominant muscular dystrophy and is caused by a deletion at chromosome 4 in 95% of patients. It is the third most common muscular dystrophy and affects 13,000 people in the UK. It causes progressive weakness of facial, neck, shoulder and limb muscles. Weakness of facial and neck muscles can cause OSA. Sleep studies in 51 consecutive patients with FSHD found sleep disordered breathing in 20 patients. Patients with FSH muscular dystrophy or muscle diseases affecting pharyngeal muscles should be screened for sleep disordered breathing routinely.

Most patients present with shoulder muscle weakness and tend to have weakness of the facial muscles with a difficulty in pronouncing words. Extra ocular and pharyngeal muscles are speared in most patients at presentation; however, with the disease progression, neck and pharyngeal muscles become weak. The extra muscular manifestations include high-frequency hearing loss (75%), retina telangiectasia (60%) and atrial arrhythmia (5%).

4. Does upper airway muscle training, strengthening or stimulation have a role in the treatment of OSA?

A study from Switzerland found that four months of upper airway muscle training by playing a didgeridoo reduced apnoeas, snoring and daytime sleepiness in non-obese patients with mild to moderate OSA. Encouraged by this study, researchers from Brazil showed that oropharyngeal exercises—exercising the tongue, soft palate and facial muscles for 30 minutes every day—led to an improvement in OSA in 16 mildly obese patients with moderate degree OSA.

German researchers attempted to train tongue muscles using electrical stimulation for 20 minutes twice a day. They found an improvement in snoring, but no effect on obstructive apnoea. Similarly, Japanese researchers attempted submental electrical stimulation following detection of apnoeas and found an improvement in some indices of sleep apnoea. It is not clear if electrical muscle stimulation caused the sleep disturbance rather than improving sleep quality.

Overall, the concept of oropharyngeal exercises is based on the assumption that pharyngeal muscles are weak or can be over-strengthened despite the lack of evidence of upper airway muscle weakness in most OSA patients. Nevertheless, lifestyle advice of regular exercise and weight loss still remains helpful.

Learning points

Upper airway muscles have an important role in keeping upper airways open during sleep.

In OSA patients, anatomically narrow upper airways increase the work of upper airway muscles and make them work harder.

It is unlikely that upper airway muscles can be strengthened/over-trained with oropharyngeal exercises; however, exercises such as playing a didgeridoo improve OSA.

Patients with neuromuscular disorders affecting upper airway muscles are at risk of OSA and should be investigated.

Further reading

Bourke SC Gibson GJ. Sleep and breathing in neuromuscular disease. Eur Respir J 2002 Jun;19(6):1194–201. Review.

Guimarães KC, Drager LF, Genta PR, Marcondes BF, Lorenzi-Filho G. Effects of oropharyngeal exercises on patients with moderate obstructive sleep apnea syndrome. Am J Respir Crit Care Med 2009 May 15;179(10):962–6.

Puhan MA, Suarez A, Lo Cascio C, Zahn A, Heitz M, Braendli O. Didgeridoo playing as alternative treatment for obstructive sleep apnoea syndrome: randomised controlled trial. BMJ 2006 Feb 4;332(7536):266–70.

Case 5
A sleepy bus driver

A 41-year-old lady was referred for an urgent assessment by the bariatric team. She gave a history of loud snoring and witnessed apnoeas. She described sleepiness and rated herself on the ESS with a rating of 21 out of 24. She had prior medical history of depression, migraines and asthma. She was prescribed asthma inhalers which she rarely used, as well as fluoxetine. She worked as a bus driver and admitted to momentary lapses of concentration when driving, although she had had no motor vehicle accidents. She regularly consumed energy drinks, as she felt these helped keep her awake.

On examination she was obese, with a BMI of 54.3. She had a crowded oropharynx with a Mallampati score of 3 and reported three episodes of tonsillitis in the previous year.

Due to her status as an occupational driver, a sleep study was performed that night. Pulse oximetry revealed a 4% dip rate of 99 events/hour with a minimum SpO_2 of 33% (Figure 5.1).

She was commenced on CPAP the next day. She had an average compliance of 6.5 hours/night on auto-titration and was commenced on a fixed pressure of 11 cm of water. When seen back at clinic, her sleepiness had resolved (ESS 2/24) and her snoring had been abolished.

She informed the Driver Vehicle Licensing Agency (DVLA) of her diagnosis and underwent regular review to ascertain the effectiveness of her CPAP treatment. In view of her large tonsils and recurrent tonsillitis, she was referred for a tonsillectomy, which was performed. Post-operative recovery was uneventful.

She subsequently underwent bariatric surgery. Post-operative recovery was uneventful. When she was seen at clinic some months after surgery,

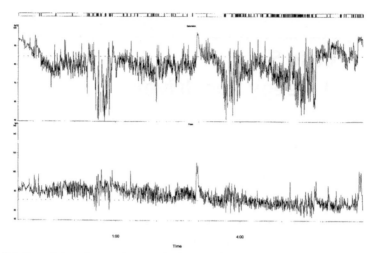

Fig. 5.1 Overnight oximetry sleep study showing frequent oxygen desaturations.

she had lost 50 kg in weight (BMI 36). She had remained on CPAP, but was finding the pressure more difficult to tolerate. A sleep study was performed off CPAP, which showed complete resolution of her sleep apnoea (4% ODI 0.65 events/hour) (Figure 5.2). Her CPAP was discontinued and the DVLA were informed of a cure of her sleep apnoea.

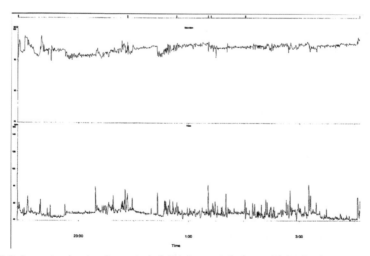

Fig. 5.2 Repeat oximetry sleep study following weight loss with bariatric surgery showing complete elimination of recurrent oxygen desaturations.

Questions

1 How is sleepiness assessed?
2 What are the post-operative risks of sleep apnoea?
3 What are the motor vehicle accident risks of sleep apnoea?

Answers

1. How is sleepiness assessed?

Sleepiness is defined as the propensity to fall asleep and should be differentiated from tiredness, which is regarded as a psychological propensity to feel fatigued. Sleepiness can be assessed by patient history as well as objective measures which may be undertaken in the sleep laboratory.

The most common measure of sleepiness used is the ESS, which is an eight-point questionnaire assessing the self-rated likelihood of falling asleep in a number of defined situations. The questionnaire has been validated against EEG markers of sleep and is the most commonly used questionnaire. It has the benefit of being self-administered and easy to use. Usually, score of >11 is regarded as showing that the patient is sleepy, and score of >15 indicates severe sleepiness. However, the scale is not perfect—for example, severely sleepy patients may avoid situations in which they are likely to fall asleep, giving an aberrantly low score, resulting in an underestimate of their sleepiness. Drivers may also be reluctant to admit to sleepiness when driving for fear of losing their licence.

The American Academy of Sleep Medicine has suggested assessing sleepiness in the history by asking the patient about falling asleep in active (e.g. having a conversation), semi-active (e.g. at the cinema) and passive (e.g. watching television) situations, and this may provide a rough guide of sleepiness.

Other questionnaires to assess sleepiness are available (Berlin sleep questionnaire, Pittsburgh sleep questionnaire), but are less frequently used. It is often useful to get a partner's estimate of sleepiness, and many clinics will routinely ask partners to attend clinic appointments and to fill in an Epworth score on their perception of their partner's sleepiness.

Sleepiness may also be measured using studies in the sleep laboratory. The multiple sleep latency time (MSLT) involves giving patients five nap opportunities in a dark, quiet room. EEG monitoring is used to confirm the onset of sleep and the mean time taken to fall asleep is taken from five sleep opportunities. An MSLT of <8 minutes is regarded as showing sleepiness. The test is mainly used to aid in the diagnosis of narcolepsy (a neurological condition causing sleepiness) and, in this case, the onset of REM sleep in at least two sleep opportunities with a mean sleep latency time of <8 minutes may be regarded as diagnostic. An overnight sleep study should be done the night before an MSLT to ensure that other sleep disorders or sleep deprivation (both of which may cause sleep onset REM) have been excluded. The test is difficult to perform and is labour intensive. It is largely carried out in specialist centres used to confirm a diagnosis of narcolepsy.

A maintenance of wakefulness test (MWT) is less well validated than MSLT. The patient has EEG monitoring and is placed in a quiet, dark room for five separate periods. In this test, the patient is given instruction to stay awake on each occasion. The Osler test is a variant of the MWT. EEG monitoring is not required. A red light is intermittently flashed at random intervals and the patient asked to press a button registering that they have seen the light. The lack of response to the light is taken as an indication that the patient has fallen asleep.

Osler and the MWT have been used mainly to ascertain the effectiveness of treatment in patients whose work is vigilance critical, e.g. to ascertain the effectiveness of CPAP treatment in heavy goods vehicle drivers. However, while improvements in MWT and Osler may be seen after treatment of sleep apnoea, there is no clear evidence that performance on a single day is related to accident risk.

2. What are the post-operative risks of sleep apnoea?

There are several case reports of patients with previously undiagnosed or unrecognized sleep apnoea going into respiratory failure after an anaesthetic. Use of anaesthetic agents may result in the loss of the usual arousal mechanism that occurs after an apnoea. Thus, patients with sleep apnoea may desaturate more profoundly and become more hypoxic after an anaesthetic.

Patients with sleep apnoea may have reduced airway calibre than those without. This may result potentially in a more difficult intubation and may be especially crucial in patients undergoing upper airway surgery who may have additional upper airway compromise due to post-operative upper airway oedema.

During an anaesthetic, there may be intra-operative atelectasis, which will result in reduction of functional residual capacity (FRC) and a resultant decrease in lung volume. Reductions in lung volume will allow the upper airway to become more collapsible and may exacerbate pre-existing sleep apnoea.

It is very difficult to perform any randomized trials on the risk of sleep apnoea in the post-operative period and much of the evidence comes from observational studies which differ widely in the surgery carried out, type of anaesthesia given and location of post-operative care (High Dependency Unit (HDU) versus ward).

As no randomized controlled data exist for this group of patients, it is difficult to make firm recommendations. Many anaesthetists will advise putting post-operative patients with sleep apnoea on to CPAP when extubated and, for this reason, prefer that patients are initiated and habituated to CPAP in the pre-operative period. Closer observations in an HDU setting may be appropriate in the post-operative period.

3. What are the motor vehicle accident risks of sleep apnoea?

There are difficulties in assessing the exact risks of patients with untreated OSA who are driving. Patients will often under-report any issues with driving for fear of losing their licence. This is particularly relevant in patients who may rely on driving for their livelihood.

Epidemiological studies have reported an increased risk of between 1.9 and 10.9 of patients with OSA having motor vehicle accidents. There is also evidence from simulator performance and vigilance testing that driving performance is impaired in untreated patients. CPAP has been shown to improve performance on both driving simulators and vigilance testing. Accident risk in OSA has been estimated to reduce by 40% in patients treated with CPAP.

Learning points

Excessive daytime sleepiness can be assessed either by using a sleepiness questionnaire, such as ESS, or objectively by measurement of MSLT or maintenance of wakefulness (MWT).

EDS due to OSA increases the risk of motor vehicle accidents.

OSA increases post-operative risks, which can be prevented by prior treatment with CPAP.

Further reading

Chung F et al. Patients with difficult airway may need referral to sleep clinics. Anaes Analg 2008;107:1543–63.

George CF. Driving and automobile crashes in patients with obstructive sleep apnoea hypopnoea syndrome. Thorax 2004;59:804–7.

Case 6
Rapid onset daytime sleep presenting as transient loss of consciousness

A 27-year-old single Asian man employed as a healthcare worker, presented to the A&E department following an episode of loss of consciousness. He was helping a patient to dress when, all of a sudden, he went blank and stopped what he was doing for about five minutes, though he could hear people shouting his name. During another episode, witnessed by his brother, whilst walking home from a mosque, he stopped walking all of a sudden, stared straight ahead and became unresponsive for about a minute, and then returned rapidly to normal. He reported four or five similar episodes over two years. He was suspected to have petit-mal seizures, but the neurologist felt that the history was not typical for epilepsy—the episodes were not associated with postictal phenomenon, automatism and orofacial movements, and were preceded by an increasing fatigue before the apparent loss of consciousness. However, complex partial seizures could not be ruled out, and an MRI head scan and EEG were requested and treatment with Lamotrigine recommended. The neurologist noted that his sleep was disturbed and of poor quality, with EDS (ESS 18/24) and he was obese. He was suspected to have OSA and referred to a sleep clinic.

His MRI head scan was normal, but showed complete occlusion of the hypopharynx at the tongue base on the sagittal view and of the oral cavity, with apposition of the tongue to the soft palate on the coronal view (Figure 6.1).

During the EEG recording, he fell asleep and the neurophysiologist found him to have frequent apnoeas. His EEG pattern rotated between

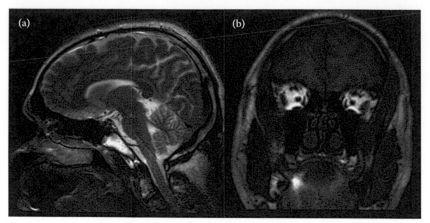

Fig. 6.1 MRI head sagittal section (a) and coronal section (b) showing complete occlusion of upper airway at the back of the tongue and soft palate.

the wake state and stage 1 sleep. His breathing cycled between periods of rapid shallow breathing and apnoeas before an abrupt arousal from stage 1 into wakefulness. Further, the apnoeic phase was associated with progressive bradycardia down to 32/min, followed by tachycardia upon arousal. An EEG was otherwise normal throughout and showed no epileptiform or focal features.

He was seen at a sleep clinic and gave a history of loud, disruptive snoring, poor quality sleep and sleep disturbance for no apparent reason, and marked daytime sleepiness, 'feeling lazy and sleepy at work'. He did not drive. He was obese, weighing 111 kg for his height of 168 cm, with a waist/hip ratio of >1, a collar size of 47 cm and an oral cavity size of 3 on the Mallampati scoring. His daytime SaO_2 were normal at 97%. A multichannel home sleep study confirmed the diagnosis of severe OSA: the AHI was 79.9 and it mainly consisted of obstructive apnoeas at 73.9%, with a mean apnoea duration of 20.7 seconds and the longest apnoea for 70.2 seconds. Apnoeas were associated with nocturnal intermittent hypoxia; the mean SaO_2 was low at 83% and he had recurrent intermittent oxygen desaturations with a SaO_2 dip rate of 94.6/hour. He spent 79.3% representing 183.4 minutes of his sleep time below SaO_2 90%. He was commenced on CPAP treatment.

Questions

1 How do you differentiate between EDS due to OSA and transient loss of consciousness due to epilepsy?

2 What does an MRI head scan show?

3 What are the effects of obstructive apnoea on the heart rate?

Answers

1. How do you differentiate between EDS due to OSA and transient loss of consciousness due to epilepsy?

EDS and falling asleep during the daytime is a common presenting feature of OSA. However, rapid onset of intense daytime sleepiness leading to sleep could be confused with transient loss of consciousness due to other causes. Transient loss of consciousness due to epilepsy is easy to recognize if associated with other features of epilepsy. The associated features are often absent in petit-mal or complex partial seizures and an EEG is required for the confirmation of the diagnosis. A normal EEG and observation of obstructed apnoea during sleep by a neurophysiologist pointed to the diagnosis of OSA. EDS is common in OSA patients and they often report falling asleep watching television, reading a book or sometimes when stopped at traffic lights while driving. However, it is unusual for OSA patients to experience intense sleepiness enough for them to fall asleep during motor activities, such as walking. EDS is mainly due to sleep disruption and poor sleep quality as a result of recurrent obstructive apnoeas.

2. What does an MRI head scan show?

A normal MRI head scan excluded a neurological cause for apparent episodes of transient loss of consciousness. However, an MRI (performed while the patient is in a lying down position) demonstrated an incidental finding of upper airway occlusion (Figure 6.1). Upper airway imaging techniques, including an MRI scan, have shown that patients with OSA have narrow upper airways when awake and sitting, which completely obstruct on lying down during sleep. Upper airway narrowing and obstruction is either located at the back of the tongue or soft palate, or can be at multiple levels. The narrow upper airway becomes narrower on lying down due to the tongue/soft palate falling back as a result of gravity. During sleep, loss of the upper airway muscle tone leads to complete or partial obstruction of the upper airway and cessation of breathing (obstructive apnoea).

3. What are the effects of obstructive apnoea on the heart rate?

Brady–tachycardia is due to autonomic changes in OSA.

During the apnoea, marked bradycardia was observed followed by tachycardia at the termination of the apnoea (Figure 6.2). Heart rate variability is a common finding in patients with OSA and a reflection of autonomic changes and hypoxia caused by obstructed breathing during sleep. The onset of apnoea results in intense vagal stimulation and bradycardia. This is similar to a diving reflex (bradycardia and apnoea on submersion in cold water). At the termination of the apnoea, an increase in sympathetic activity causes tachycardia. The autonomic changes are also thought to contribute to high prevalence of (brady and tachy) arrhythmias and changes in blood pressure in OSA. Heart rate variability can be detected as brady–tachycardia on ECG, or RR variability on a 24 ECG recording (Holter monitoring). In fact, RR variability is so characteristic of OSA that Holter monitoring can provide indirect support for the diagnosis of OSA.

Learning points

Apparent transient loss of consciousness can be due to intense daytime sleepiness in OSA.

Imaging techniques such as MRI head show upper airway obstruction at the tongue base and/or soft palate level in OSA.

OSA patients have brady–tachycardia during sleep due to autonomic changes.

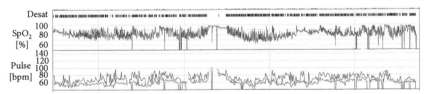

Fig. 6.2 Sleep pulse oximetry (SaO$_2$ and pulse rate) recording showing variation in pulse rate (heart rate) variable associated with recurrent oxygen desaturations due to OSA.

Further reading

Guilleminault C, Brooks SN. Excessive daytime sleepiness: a challenge for the practising neurologist. Brain 2001 Aug;124(Pt 8):1482–91. Review.

Gula LJ, Krahn AD, Skanes AC, Yee R, Klein GJ. Clinical relevance of arrhythmias during sleep: guidance for clinicians. Heart 2004 Mar;90(3):347–52. Review.

Schwab RJ. Imaging for the snoring and sleep apnea patient. Dent Clin North Am 2001 Oct;45(4):759–96. Review.

Case 7
Unexplained breathlessness and pulmonary arterial hypertension in an obese man

A 78-year-old obese Indian man, an ex-smoker with a history of non-insulin diabetes mellitus and hypertension, presented with worsening exertional breathlessness four years ago. He was seen by a cardiologist and found to have rate-controlled atrial fibrillation, mild mitral regurgitation with a dilated left atrium, good left ventricular ejection fraction (55%) and a high estimated pulmonary arterial pressure of 60 mmHg. A myocardial perfusion scan confirmed good LV function and mild reversible ischemia. He was treated with warfarin and frusemide. His exertional breathlessness and pulmonary hypertension could not be explained on the basis of the cardiac findings and he was referred to a respiratory physician for further investigations. His pulmonary function tests showed mild restrictive impairment FEV 1.5 litre (1.9 predicted) and FVC 2.0 (2.8 predicted) and the CT PA angiogram showed no evidence of pulmonary embolism or pulmonary parenchymal abnormality. He had mild eventration of the right diaphragm.

His breathlessness worsened over the next two years with a reduction in exercise tolerance to 30 yards on the flat. His repeat CT chest scan showed mild bronchiectasis and small airway disease, and no change in diaphragmatic eventration. His pulmonary function tests showed no change in extrathoracic pulmonary restriction, but he had mild airflow obstruction. His diaphragmatic function test—maximum expiratory and inspiratory pressures at the mouth (PEmax and PImax)—were normal and arterial blood gases showed mild hypoxia without any hypercapnia or acidosis. He was suspected to have OSA when he reported feeling sleepy during the daytime and was referred to a sleep clinic.

He lived and slept alone, but his friends/family members reported snoring without witnessed apnoea when he visited them. He slept well, apart from waking up two to three times to pass urine. He was sleepy during the daytime on watching television or sitting inactive. He was retired and did not drive. He reported no reduced concentration or impaired memory. He had put on about 5 kg in weight over the last five years. He was obese (BMI 36).

His overnight oximetry sleep study confirmed OSA—his 4% oxygen desaturation dip rate was 36/hour with a characteristic sawtooth pattern. It showed nocturnal hypoxia—mean SaO_2 was 89% and total sleep time (TST) below SaO_2 90% was 69%. A repeat sleep study on CPAP after a week on CPAP showed a normal dip rate of 1.38 and an improved but persistent nocturnal hypoxia with mean SaO_2 89.42%. He was commenced on overnight oxygen at a flow rate of 1 litre/minute via a CPAP mask. A repeat echocardiogram a year later showed no evidence of pulmonary arterial hypertension.

Questions

1 What was the explanation for the breathlessness?

2 What was the explanation for the pulmonary arterial hypertension?

3 Why did he have nocturia and urinary frequency?

Answers

1. What was the explanation for the breathlessness?

His breathlessness was probably due to obesity. Obese subjects, particularly smokers, are at a much higher risk of cardiorespiratory problems and should be investigated for conditions such as ischemic heart disease and airflow obstruction when they present with breathlessness. However, in the absence of cardiorespiratory abnormality, obesity may be the only explanation for breathlessness. Surveys have shown that 80% of obese subjects report breathlessness on exertion and one third of non-insulin dependent diabetes mellitus patients had troublesome breathlessness. Obese smokers are breathless even at rest because the effect of a minor degree of airflow obstruction on breathlessness is exaggerated.

Obesity often causes mild pulmonary restriction due to a large amount of extrathoracic and abdominal fat causing a reduction in chest wall compliance and diaphragmatic excursion. They also have associated airflow obstruction due to smoking or obesity itself. They may have weak respiratory muscles due to fatty infiltration. The combination of these abnormalities increases the work of breathing, both at rest and on exertion, and causes breathlessness. The abdominal visceral obesity causes ventilation–perfusion mismatch at the lung bases and a mild degree of hypoxia at rest which worsens on exertion or lying down flat.

2. What was the explanation for the pulmonary arterial hypertension?

Chronic intermittent nocturnal hypoxia as a result of undiagnosed OSA is a likely explanation for raised pulmonary arterial pressure. Impaired LV diastolic function and left atrial enlargement may have also contributed to the raised pulmonary arterial pressures.

Hypoxia (acute or chronic) is a well-recognized factor in the causation of pulmonary arterial hypertension. Rodents, when exposed to brief, intermittent hypoxia to mimic OSA, developed pulmonary vascular remodelling and sustained pulmonary hypertension and right ventricular hypertrophy within a few weeks. In OSA, recurrent intermittent arterial oxygen desaturations are associated with an increase in pulmonary artery pressures. Approximately one-third of patients with OSA have a modest degree of pulmonary arterial hypertension in the absence of a cardiopulmonary cause. It is more common in obese patients who have severe nocturnal hypoxia and low daytime paO_2. However, raised PAP is rarely associated with right-sided heart failure. It improves/normalizes with CPAP. OSA should be considered as a cause of unexplained/incidental raised pulmonary arterial hypertension.

3. Why did he have nocturia and urinary frequency?

OSA patients often report nocturia and urinary frequency. This is often thought to be due to benign prostatic hypertrophy (BPH) or diabetes mellitus. It has been suggested that nocturia in BPH may be due to associated OSA. A recent community study found patients with BPH and nocturia had a much higher risk of OSA than patients without BPH. Furthermore, nocturia was found to be a good predictor of OSA. Nocturia in OSA is due to an increase in secretion of atrial natriuretic peptide (ANP) that encourages diuresis. The ANP levels return to normal and nocturia often improves with treatment of OSA with CPAP.

Learning points

Obesity increases the work of breathing and impairs respiratory function and can cause breathlessness.

Chronic intermittent hypoxia due to undiagnosed obstructive apnoea can cause pulmonary arterial hypertension which may resolve with treatment of OSA.

OSA should be considered as a possible cause of nocturia even in patients with diabetes mellitus and benign prostatic hypertrophy.

Further reading

Arias MA, Garcia-Rio F, Alonso-Fernandez A, Martinez I, Villamor J. Pulmonary hypertension in obstructive sleep apnoea: effects of continuous positive airway pressure: a randomized, controlled cross-over study. Eur Heart J 2006;27:1106–13.

Gibson GJ. Obesity, respiratory function and breathlessness. Thorax 2000 Aug;55 (Suppl 1):S41–4. Review.

Romero E, Krakow B, Haynes P, Ulibarri V. Nocturia and snoring: predictive symptoms for obstructive sleep apnea. Sleep Breath 2010 Dec;14(4):337–43.

Case 8
Post-operative apnoeas and hypoxia due to undiagnosed OSA

A 66-year-old man, a smoker of a 50 pack year with a history of hypertension and angioplasty for myocardial infarction, had two transient ischaemic attacks and was found to have 70% stenosis of the left internal carotid artery. He underwent a left-sided carotid endarterectomy. During post-operative period he had multiple episodes of apnoea associated with low oxygen saturations and referred to a sleep clinic. He had moderate bruising around the left neck wound following surgery. He snored heavily and had witnessed apnoea, according to his wife. He felt tired and sleepy during the daytime (ESS 14/24) and often nodded off at meetings working as a financial advisor—he did not drive. He was morbidly obese with a BMI of 51.3, neck size of 50 cm and a crowded oral cavity (Mallampati score of 4). He had evidence of airflow obstruction on spirometry lung function tests: FEV_1 1.7 litre (55% of predicted) and FVC 2.5 litre. His visilab sleep study consisting of overnight audio-video monitoring with oximetry confirmed the diagnosis of severe OSA. The oximetry showed characteristic repetitive SaO_2 desaturations with a dip rate of 39.31/hour and nocturnal hypoxia with mean SaO_2 of 83.62%. Observation of the video recording during desaturation confirmed loud snoring following by prolonged obstructive apnoeas. His daytime SaO_2 on air were normal at 94%.

He was treated with CPAP at a fixed pressure of 9 cm of water delivered via a nasal CPAP mask. CPAP was effective in correcting his OSA, with a reduction in SaO_2 dips to 3.91 hours and nocturnal hypoxia persisted—mean SaO_2 86.62%. His objective CPAP compliance was satisfactory. His sleep quality improved and he felt less tired and sleepy during the daytime (ESS 4/12). He had a reduced exercise tolerance of half a flight of stairs and was unable to lose any weight, despite an improvement in his daytime symptoms. He was referred to a bariatric service; however, he refused to have bariatric surgery or consider dietary interventions. He had frequent admissions to hospital because of acute hypercapnic respiratory failure following pneumonia and a lower respiratory tract infection, and required prolonged invasive ventilation and a prolonged stay on the intensive care unit. The CPAP was changed to bi-level positive airway pressure (BiPAP), and he had no further admissions to hospital and noticed an improvement in sleep, daytime sleepiness and exercise tolerance.

Questions

1 What are the peri-operative risks and peri-operative complications of undiagnosed/untreated OSA?

2 How can you prevent these complications?

3 Is there any difference in the risks between different types of surgery in patients with OSA?

Answers

1. What are the peri-operative risks and peri-operative complications of undiagnosed/untreated OSA?

OSA remains undiagnosed in 80% of the population. Patients with undiagnosed/untreated OSA are at an increased risk of peri-operative respiratory complications. During the pre-operative period, use of pre-operative sedation and upper airway muscles relaxation can precipitate OSA and hypoxia. Patients with OSA have narrow upper airways and are at a higher risk of difficult (tracheal) intubation. Prolonged apnoea during the post-operative period while recovering from a general anaesthesia can cause respiratory distress and respiratory arrest. This may need re-intubation or an emergency tracheostomy. It is known that anaesthetic agents reduce the tone of pharyngeal musculature, depress ventilation, diminish ventilatory response to carbon dioxide and also abolish arousals from sleep. Moreover, trauma from airway manipulation, drugs and pain can affect sleep architecture and regulation of the upper airway muscles in the post-operative period.

2. How can you prevent these complications?

Anaesthetists have a key role in identifying patients at an increased risk of OSA. Simple questionnaire-based screening or upper airway assessment at the pre-anaesthetic check can identify patients at an increased risk of OSA. If the assessment suggests a high risk of obstructive apnoea, they should have further sleep investigations. Identification of difficult airways at the pre-anaesthetic check-up or before intubation can help the anaesthetist plan for the management of difficult airways. Careful respiratory monitoring during the post-operative period and early intervention with non-invasive ventilator support oxygen, CPAP or BiPAP can reduce post-operative risk.

Patients undergoing bariatric surgery for morbid obesity have a very high prevalence (up to 70%) of OSA. A routine screening and assessment including a sleep study has been suggested for such a

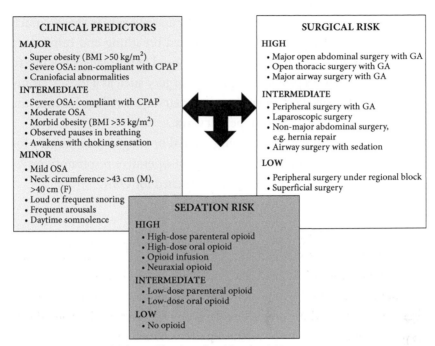

CLINICAL PREDICTORS

MAJOR
- Super obesity (BMI >50 kg/m^2)
- Severe OSA: non-compliant with CPAP
- Craniofacial abnormalities

INTERMEDIATE
- Severe OSA: compliant with CPAP
- Moderate OSA
- Morbid obesity (BMI >35 kg/m^2)
- Observed pauses in breathing
- Awakens with choking sensation

MINOR
- Mild OSA
- Neck circumference >43 cm (M), >40 cm (F)
- Loud or frequent snoring
- Frequent arousals
- Daytime somnolence

SURGICAL RISK

HIGH
- Major open abdominal surgery with GA
- Open thoracic surgery with GA
- Major airway surgery with GA

INTERMEDIATE
- Peripheral surgery with GA
- Laparoscopic surgery
- Non-major abdominal surgery, e.g. hernia repair
- Airway surgery with sedation

LOW
- Peripheral surgery under regional block
- Superficial surgery

SEDATION RISK

HIGH
- High-dose parenteral opioid
- High-dose oral opioid
- Opioid infusion
- Neuraxial opioid

INTERMEDIATE
- Low-dose parenteral opioid
- Low-dose oral opioid

LOW
- No opioid

Fig. 8.1 A suggested risk stratification algorithm for OSA.
Source: Reproduced from BMJ Case Reports, Weinberg L, et al, 2013, with permission from BMJ Publishing Group Ltd.

high-risk group of patients. Furthermore, it has been suggested that this group of patients with OSA should be established on CPAP for at least four weeks prior to surgery. A multi-disciplinary pre-operative assessment, including respiratory, prior to bariatric surgery may achieve further reduction in the risk of post-operative complications (Figure 8.1).

3. Is there any difference in the risks between different types of surgery in patients with OSA?

Patients with OSA are at double the risk of post-operative respiratory complications, even after routine knee or hip replacement surgery, than patients without OSA. This may be due to a direct effect of OSA on post-operative respiratory complications or associated morbidity such as obesity, hypertension and diabetes mellitus.

However, patients undergoing upper airways surgery have a much higher risk of post-operative obstructed breathing and respiratory complications. They may have undiagnosed or untreated OSA due to an upper airways problem requiring surgery such as a tonsillectomy for large tonsils. Post-operative upper airways swelling/haematoma may further obstruct the upper airways.

Similarly, patients undergoing palatal or tongue base surgery for snoring may be at a higher risk of post-operative respiratory problems, particularly if they were not screened for OSA.

Learning points

Undiagnosed OSA may present as post-operative apnoeas and hypoxia.

Undiagnosed OSA is associated with an increased risk of peri-operative respiratory complications.

Screening for OSA with a sleep questionnaire or upper airways assessment at a pre-anaesthetic check can identify patients at risk of OSA.

OSA patients at high risk of post-operative complications, such as morbidly obese patients with cardiovascular co-morbidity, should have a sleep study and be established on CPAP prior to surgery.

Further reading

Adesanya AO, Lee W, Greilich NB, Joshi GP. Perioperative management of obstructive sleep apnea. Chest 2010 Dec;138(6):1489–98.

den Herder C, Schmeck J, Appelboom DJ, de Vries N. Risks of general anaesthesia in people with obstructive sleep apnoea. BMJ 2004 Oct 23;329(7472):955–9. Review.

Weinberg L, Houli N, Nikfarjam M. Improving outcomes for pancreatic cancer: radical surgery with patient-tailored, surgery-specific advanced haemodynamic monitoring. BMJ Case Rep 2013 Apr 30;2013.

Case 9
Polycythemia got better with CPAP

A 56-year-old man, a retired insurance underwriter, was referred by a haematologist to establish if his polycythemia was due to nocturnal hypoxia as a result of sleep apnoea. His haemoglobin and red cell mass remained elevated, despite venesection. He was a smoker (20 per day) and known to have chronic obstructive pulmonary disease (COPD), but his exercise tolerance was more than a mile and spirometry showed moderately severe airflow obstruction (FEV$_1$ 53% of predicted, FEV$_1$/FVC 61%) with no significant reversibility.

He had put on weight after his retirement and felt sleepy during the daytime; he fell asleep on public transport on several occasions. His ESS was high at 16/24. His wife noted that he stopped breathing during his sleep. He snored loudly enough for his wife to wear earplugs or sleep in a separate room. He was plethoric and obese (BMI 30) with a neck size of 44.5 cm. His pulse was regular at 72/minute and blood pressure was normal at 125/85 mmHg. He had a widespread wheeze on auscultation of his chest.

A PSG confirmed severe OSA.

Respiratory monitoring showed frequent obstructed apnoeas (263 episodes of complete cessation of breathing for >10 seconds) and hypopnoeas (203 episodes of 50% reduction in respiratory effort for >10 seconds) with an AHI of 62.3 (number of apnoeas and hypopnoeas per hour of sleep). The average duration of apnoeas was 31 seconds and hypopnoeas 23 seconds, and the longest apnoea lasted for 138 seconds and hypopnoea 86 seconds.

Sleep monitoring demonstrated that respiratory disturbance was due to recurrent obstructive apnoea/hypopnoeas that caused disturbed and poor quality sleep. He woke up from sleep every two minutes with an EEG arousal index of 30/hour and poor sleep quality with very little dream sleep: REM sleep for 16.3 minutes only. Non-rapid eye movement (NREM) sleep consisted of light sleep (stages 1 and 2) for 164.7 minutes and deep sleep (stages 3 and 4) for 271 minutes.

Oxygen saturation (SaO$_2$) monitoring with pulse oximetry showed that apnoeas and hypopnoeas resulted in intermittent nocturnal hypoxia. There was 54/hour transient reduction in SaO$_2$ (>4% from baseline): SaO$_2$ desaturation dip rate, mean SaO$_2$ during sleep was low at 76.59% and 90% of TST spent below SaO$_2$ of 90% (TST <SaO$_2$ 90%).

His OSA was treated with CPAP at 8 cm of water delivered to the upper airways via a nasal mask. He noticed a marked improvement in his sleep quality and woke up feeling fresh, with an improvement in daytime sleepiness and a reduction in daytime sleepiness (ESS of 9/24 compared to 16/24). His self-reported CPAP compliance was six nights a week and seven hours each night. Repeat sleep study on CPAP (CPAP sleep study) showed normalization of AHI to 5.3 from a baseline AHI of 62.3. This was associated with a reduction and improvement in sleep quality and sleep disturbance. The arousal index was 9.4/hour compared to a baseline of 30/hour, and REM sleep duration increased to 148 minutes from 16.3 minutes and with no change in stage 3 and stage 4 NREM sleep duration. There was a marked improvement in the nocturnal hypoxia: mean SaO$_2$ improved to 90.92% from 76.59%, dip rate reduced to 16.17 from 54.36 and TST <90% to 2 hours and 2 minutes.

He did not require further venesection to maintain his haemoglobin within the normal range.

Questions

1 What are the criteria for the diagnosis of OSA?
2 How does OSA affect sleep?
3 What is the effect of OSA on respiration during sleep?
4 What is the effect of CPAP on sleep and respiration in OSA?

Answers

1. What are the criteria for the diagnosis of OSA?

In OSA, upper airway obstruction during sleep causes recurrent apnoeas and hypopnoeas. More than five apnoeas/hypopnoeas per hour: AHI >5 confirms the diagnosis of OSA.

Upper airway obstruction during sleep causes loud disruptive snoring and apnoeas. Confirmation of the diagnosis of OSA requires a sleep study for the measurement of the number of obstructive apnoeas and hypopnoeas per hour during sleep: known as the AHI. Apnoeas and hypopnoeas are detected by the measurement of oral and nasal airflow: complete cessation of airflow (breath) for 10 seconds or more is apnoea and 50% reduction in airflow is hypopnoea. The apnoeas and hypopnoeas are further characterized either as obstructive or central by measurement of respiratory effort (chest wall and abdominal respiratory movements). In OSA, respiratory effort persists, but it is absent in central apnoea (Figure 9.1). A total of more than five apnoeas plus hypopnoeas per hour is used as a cut-off for the diagnosis of OSA, though many of the symptomatic OSA

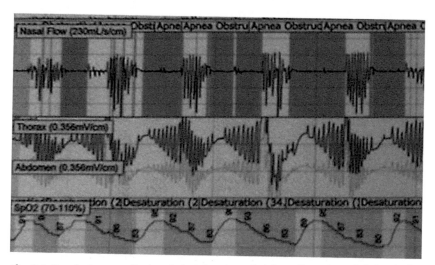

Fig. 9.1 Respiratory monitoring during sleep: nasal airflow, thoracic and abdominal wall movements, and oxygen saturation (SpO$_2$) showing prolonged obstructive apnoeas (cessation of airflow) but persistent thoraco-abdominal wall movement associated with SaO$_2$ desaturations.

patients have a much higher AHI. The presence of symptoms such as EDS in patients with AHI >5 is required to diagnose obstructive sleep apnoea syndrome (OSAS).

2. How does OSA affect sleep?

Apnoeas and hypopnoeas during sleep result in recurrent arousals, sleep fragmentation and poor quality sleep.

Some OSA patients have disturbed sleep and wake up frequently from sleep. They wake up either for no apparent reason and visit the toilet to pass urine, or wake up with a sore/dry throat, gasping for breath or choking. Others report sleeping through the night for a sufficient number of hours, but wake up unrefreshed, tired and fatigued.

Sleep quality, duration and disturbance can be measured by recording an EEG, eye movement with an electroculogram (EOG) and chin/leg muscle tone with an electromyogram (EMG). These measurements provide the amount of time spent in light sleep (NREM stages 1 and 2), deep sleep (NREM stages 3 and 4 slow wave sleep) and dream sleep (REM sleep) (Figure 9.2). The refreshing quality

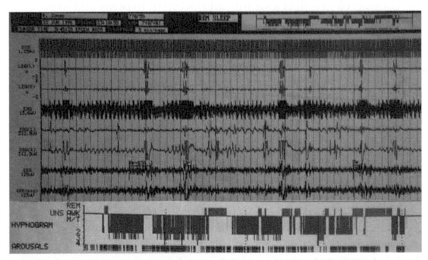

Fig. 9.2 Upper panel: a five-minute epoch of sleep monitoring during REM sleep (top to bottom: EEG, left and right leg and chin muscle, EMG, left and right electroculogram, and two EEGs) showing arousal on EEG channels associated with legs' EMG activity. Lower panel showing hypnogram with recurrent arousals.

to sleep is mainly due to slow wave and dream sleep. However, obstructive apnoeas are most common and prolonged during deep and dream sleep, and recurrent arousal results in poor quality sleep (light sleep). The measurement of the number of arousals/hour and relative duration spent during different stages of sleep (hypnogram) helps to establish sleep duration, efficiency and quality.

3. **What is the effect of OSA on respiration during sleep?**
Apnoeas and hypopnoeas during sleep result in recurrent nocturnal SaO_2 desaturation and chronic intermittent nocturnal hypoxia.

Patients with OSA have a recurrent drop in SaO_2 during sleep. A minimum drop in SaO_2 by 4% from the baseline is equated to each apnoea/hypopnoea. However, prolonged apnoea and hypopnoeas, particularly during deep and dream sleep, result in a marked drop in SaO_2 by 20% or more. Intermittent nocturnal hypoxia as a result of the effect of recurrent apnoeas and hypopnoeas can be quantified by measuring not only the number of 4% drops in SaO_2 per hour— SaO_2 dip rate—but also mean SaO_2 and TST spent below SaO_2 of 90%. Low mean SaO_2 <88% and TST of 30% below SaO_2 of 90% is considered to reflect a significant nocturnal hypoxia and hypoventilation. Patients with undiagnosed and untreated OSA have chronic intermittent hypoxia. Many of the adverse consequences of OSA, including polycythemia, are thought to be related to nocturnal hypoxia. It is likely that secondary polycythemia was due to chronic nocturnal hypoxia in the patient in this case, though contribution of the associated risk factors, such as COPD and smoking, could not be excluded.

4. **What is the effect of CPAP on sleep and respiration in OSA?**
CPAP reverses the abnormalities mentioned here and is the most effective treatment of OSA.

CPAP abolishes apnoea and hypopnoeas including snoring, corrects intermittent nocturnal hypoxia and restores sleep quality to normal.

Learning points

In OSA, upper airway obstruction during sleep causes recurrent apnoeas and hypopnoeas. More than five apnoeas/hypopnoeas per hour: AHI >5 confirms the diagnosis of OSA.

Apnoeas and hypopnoeas during sleep result in recurrent arousals, sleep fragmentation and poor quality sleep.

Apnoea and hypopnoeas during sleep result in recurrent SaO_2 desaturation and chronic intermittent hypoxia.

CPAP reverses these abnormalities and is the most effective treatment of OSA.

Further reading

McNicholas WT. Diagnosis of obstructive sleep apnea in adults. Proc Am Thorac Soc 2008;5:154–60.

National Institute of Health and Clinical Excellence (NICE). Continuous positive airway pressure for the treatment of obstructive sleep apnoea/hypopnoea syndrome. Health Technology Appraisal. NICE Technology Appraisal guidance 139 March 2008.

Scottish Intercollegiate Guidelines Network (SIGN). Management of obstructive sleep apnoea/hypopnoea syndrome in adults. Scottish Intercollegiate Guidelines Network. 2003. ISBN 1 899893 33 4

Case 10
Hyperphagia and sleep disorder in Prader-Willi Syndrome

A 22-year-old obese man with a diagnosis of Prader-Willi Syndrome was suspected to have OSA by an endocrinologist. His mother reported that he had loud, disruptive snoring and was always sleepy during the daytime—his ESS score was 17/24 (Figure 10.1). He weighed 149.2 kg for his height of 165.4 cm, but his collar size was normal at 35 cm. He was diagnosed to have Prader-Willi Syndrome at the age of 3 weeks on the basis of clinical features of almond-shaped eyes, a triangular mouth and hypotonia. The diagnosis was later confirmed at the age of 5 years with a genetic test showing deletion on chromosome 15. During puberty, he had genital hypoplasia, gynaecomastia and low testosterone levels. He was treated with testosterone and gonadotropins. His weight was 93.7 kg and his height 159.1 cm at the age of 18 years, but he put on 40 kg in weight over the next year and a half due to uncontrollable hyperphagia (Figure 10.2). His mother had to keep food locked away at home and his employer at the supermarket kept him away from the food section. He weighed 131.1 kg for his height of 165 cm at age 19 years. He also developed insulin resistance and was treated with metformin.

The visilab sleep study (audio-video sleep monitoring with oximetry) confirmed mild sleep apnoea. He was treated with a custom-made mandibular advancement splint (MAS) which eliminated snoring (his brother was able to sleep undisturbed in the next room). His sleep quality improved with a reduction in daytime tiredness, but his ESS remained high. Treatment with stimulant modafinil was considered but not prescribed, as he had stopped working and did not drive. He remained compliant with MAS with an improvement in sleep apnoea symptoms,

Even if you haven't done some of these things recently, try to work out how they would have affected you.

Use the following scale to choose the most appropriate number for each situation:

   0   would never doze

   1   slight chance of dozing

   2   moderate chance of dozing

   3   high chance of dozing

SITUATION	CHANCE OF DOZING
Sitting and reading	2
Watching television	3
Sitting, inactive in a public place, e.g. theatre/meeting	3
Sitting, as a passenger in a car for an hour without a break	3
Lying down to rest in the afternoon when circumstances permit	3
Sitting and talking to someone	0
Sitting quietly after a lunch without alcohol	3
In a car, while stopped for a few minutes in the traffic	0

TOTAL SCORE : ....17....

Fig. 10.1 ESS in a patient with Prader-Willi Syndrome.

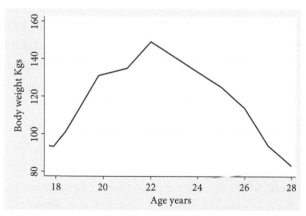

Fig. 10.2 Graph showing change in body weight (BMI) in patients with Prader-Willi Syndrome.

and lost 25 kg in weight with a combination of dietary restriction and exercise over the next three years. He lost further weight with the appetite suppressing agent rimonabant over the next year. His MAS broke, but he had no snoring or disturbed sleep despite not using his splint for a year. A repeat sleep study at the age of 28 years, when he had lost a total of 57 kg and weighed 83.2 kg, showed no evidence of sleep apnoea and he was discharged from the clinic.

Questions

1 What are the common causes of obesity in children?
2 What is the explanation for hyperphagia and obesity in patients with Prader-Willi Syndrome?
3 How common is sleep apnoea in patients with Prader-Willi Syndrome?

Answers

1. **What are the common causes of obesity in children?**

   In the UK, approximately 10% of school children in reception (5–6 years) and 20% in Year 6 (10–11 years) are obese and at risk of developing obesity-related problems. OSA has been reported to occur in up to 60% of obese children and adolescents. Obesity in most children is due to an unhealthy lifestyle—excessive eating and lack of exercise. However, in a few, it can be due to endocrine/genetic disorders. It can be due to endocrine problems, such as Cushing's syndrome and hypothyroidism. Prader-Willi Syndrome is the commonest hereditary cause of obesity. It is seen in 1 out of 20,000 children. In most, it is due to non-inherited (*de novo*) mutation in paternally derived chromosome 15.

2. **What is the explanation for hyperphagia and obesity in patient with Prader-Willi Syndrome?**

   Patients with Prader-Willi Syndrome go through different stages of feeding/eating problems. During infancy, an inability to suck effectively makes them undernourished and lose weight, with no further difficulties in feeding during childhood. This is followed by hyperphagia and an insatiable appetite during adolescence, leading to morbid obesity.

   Hyperphagia is due to hypothalamic dysfunction causing decreased satiety, an increased reward to food and increased hunger. They have high levels of leptin and ghrelin which should lead to satiety and decreased food intake. However, patients with hypothalamic dysfunction fail to respond to these feedback mechanisms to control appetite. Hyperphagia is best managed with a strict controlled diet and reduced access to food.

3. **How common is sleep apnoea in patients with Prader-Willi Syndrome?**

   Respiratory problems during sleep are very common in adult patients with Prader-Willi Syndrome—one study found 95% of patients with the syndrome had OSA. It is mainly due to obesity; however, associated hypotonia and reduced respiratory drive also contribute to nocturnal hypoventilation seen in many of these patients. Marked daytime sleepiness (hypersomnia) is due to a combination of OSA and hypothalamic dysfunction, and may persist despite treatment of OSA. However, treatment of OSA with CPAP has the potential of improving neurocognitive function.

Learning points

Childhood obesity is common and rising. In most children, it is due to an unhealthy lifestyle but, in a few, it could be due to genetic and endocrine causes.

Prader-Willi Syndrome is the commonest genetic cause of OSA.

Most patients with Prader-Willi Syndrome have OSA.

Hypersomnia due to hypothalamic syndrome may persist despite treatment of OSA with CPAP.

Further reading

Butler MG. Prader-Willi Syndrome: obesity due to genomic imprinting. Current Genomics 2011;12:204–15.

correcting his sleep apnoea. He remains obese due to hyperphagia and hypersomnolence, despite correction of sleep apnoea due to hypothalamic syndrome as a result of the brain injury during childhood.

Questions

1 What is the role of hypothalamus in control of appetite and sleep?
2 How is our sleep rhythm generated and controlled?
3 What is hypothalamic syndrome?

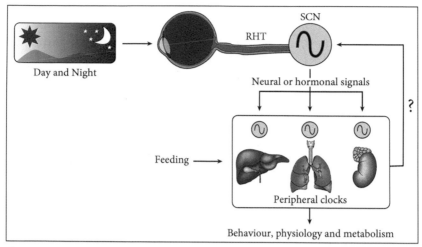

Fig. 11.2 Components of the mammalian circadian clock system. Changes in light due to the day/night cycle are directly detected by the eyes. The light information is transported to the SCN in the anterior hypothalamus by the retinohypothalamic tract (RHT). The SCN functions as a master circadian oscillator where circadian rhythmicity is generated. The generated circadian rhythmicity is converted into output pathways that control the behaviour, physiology and metabolism of the organisms. These environmental signals, core circadian oscillator and output rhythms are three basic components of the circadian clock system.
Source: Reproduced with permission from Ilmin Kwon, Han Kyoung Choe, Gi Hoon Son and Kyungjin Kim, Mammalian Molecular Clocks, Exp Neurobiol. Mar 2011; 20(1): 18–28, distributed under Creative Commons License 3.0.

temperature and hormone secretion, is approximately a day (circadian rhythms), with peaks and troughs at different times of a day. This accounts for us feeling sleepy at certain times of the day—late in the evening or afternoons. The natural sleep cycle is of 25 hours' duration. However, neurons in the core of the SCN are sensitive to light and contain melatonin receptors which respond to external clues such as light and clock time. Light stimulates receptors in the retina and via the retinohypothalamic tract controls melatonin secretions—switched off by light and on by darkness. This helps to override the natural sleep cycle rhythm of 25 hours and reset it to 24 hours' duration. There is fine coordination (synchronization) between different biological rhythms, for example a change in our body temperature is synchronized with sleep cycles—sleep onset is

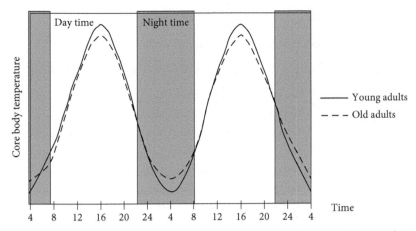

Fig. 11.3 Showing changes in core body temperature during the normal sleep cycle in young and old adults.
Source: Wen-Chun Liao, Ming-Jang Chiu, and Carol A. Landi, A warm footbath before bedtime and sleep in older Taiwanese with sleep disturbance, Res Nurs Health. 2008 October; 31(5): 514–528, with permission from John Wiley & Sons Ltd.

associated with a fall in temperature and a rise during wakefulness (Figure 11.3).

3. What is hypothalamic syndrome?

The hypothalamus controls endocrine, neurological and autonomic functions and biological rhythms. Damage to the hypothalamus can result in a variable combination of loss of endocrine function, neurological problems, autonomic dysfunction and alternation in biological rhythms—hypothalamic syndrome. The exact clinical features of the syndrome depend on the extent and site of damage to the hypothalamus. They have clinical features of endocrine (pituitary) deficiency associated with non-endocrine features, such as abnormal behaviour, hypersomnia, eating disorders, hyperphagia and loss of thermoregulation. In adults, hypothalamic damage is often due to a tumour, such as craniopharyngioma, granulomatous inflammation from sarcoidosis and cerebrovascular stroke. In children, it is often due to congenital disorder/genetic syndrome. Head injury or a history of cranial surgery is one of the common causes of hypothalamic syndrome in both children and adults.

Learning points

The hypothalamus regulates sleep and appetite.

Hypothalamic damage can cause loss of satiety and uncontrollable eating and obesity.

OSA contributes to morbidity from hypothalamic syndrome.

Further reading

Guftar Shaikh M. Hypothalamic dysfunction (hypothalamic syndromes) 2.4.1 Oxford Textbook of Endocrinology and Diabetes (2nd ed.) Edited by JAH Wass, PM Stewart, SA Amiel, MC Davies. Oxford University Press. 2011.

Saper CB, Scammell TE, Lu J. Hypothalamic regulation of sleep and circadian rhythms. Nature October 2005;437:1257–1263.

Case 12
Collapsed in a café: acute respiratory failure

A 46-year-old morbidly obese man went to a café and ordered a breakfast. He collapsed and slumped on a table before breakfast arrived. Paramedics on the scene found him unresponsive and took to him to the Accident and Emergency as an 'unwell adult'. His Glasgow Coma Scale (GCS) was 8, temperature 37°C, blood pressure 148/81 mmHg and respiratory rate 28/min. His plasma glucose was elevated at 12.3 mmol/l and other blood tests showed a mildly elevated white cell count of 13.6 and C-reactive protein (CRP) of 6 (normal >5), but urea, creatinine, electrolytes and liver function tests were are all normal. ECG showed normal sinus rhythm and troponin was normal. He received high flow oxygen at 15 l/min via a rebreathing mask and arterial blood gases (ABG) showed pH 7.209, pCO_2 10.5 kPa, pO_2 12.5 kPa and HCO_3 31.1 mmol/l—consistent with acute on chronic hypercapnic respiratory failure. His portable chest X-ray was difficult to interpret (Figure 12.1), but showed no evidence of collapse/consolidation or pulmonary oedema. He was intubated and ventilated, and a CT head scan performed on the way to the intensive therapy unit (ITU) was normal. A probable diagnosis of viral/bacterial meningoencephalitis was made and treated with acyclovir and cefotriaxone while awaiting further investigations.

His mother was contacted, who informed that he had had speech and hearing impairments since birth, but was otherwise in good health and had had a sleep study for sleep apnoea done at another hospital a few weeks previously (Figure 12.2). She described that he had experienced breathing difficulties and choking during sleep for a number of years and was often sleepy during the daytime—he was found twice on the street by police in

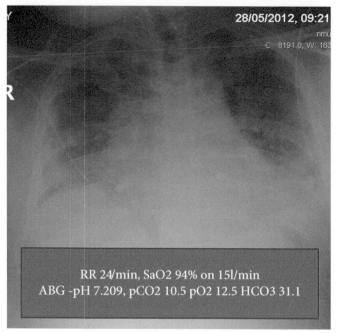

28/05/2012, 09:21

RR 24/min, SaO2 94% on 15l/min
ABG -pH 7.209, pCO2 10.5 pO2 12.5 HCO3 31.1

Fig. 12.1 Difficult to interpret portable chest radiograph, but showing no collapse consolidation or pulmonary oedema in patient with acute hypercapnic respiratory failure.

a drunken state, but he never drank alcohol. His sleep study was retrieved and showed severe OSA with marked nocturnal hypoxia. He was waiting for a trial of CPAP, but could not be contacted on the telephone.

His comatose state and acute hypercapnic respiratory failure were attributed to severe OSA associated with nocturnal hypoventilation (Obesity Hypoventilation Syndrome). He was extubated and established on CPAP. He tolerated CPAP well, slept well and was less sleepy during the day. A repeat sleep study on CPAP showed an improvement in sleep apnoea and nocturnal hypoxia. He was stepped down to the high dependency unit (HDU) and discharged on the fourth day. He was reviewed in the sleep clinic a week later. He weighed 175 kg for his height of 171 cm and a neck size of 46 cm, with a grade three size oral cavity on the Mallampati scoring system. His spirometry lung function showed FVC of 3.76 (83% of predicted), FEV1 3.69 (84% of predicted) and FEV1/FVC 82%. His daytime resting SaO_2 were normal at 94%.

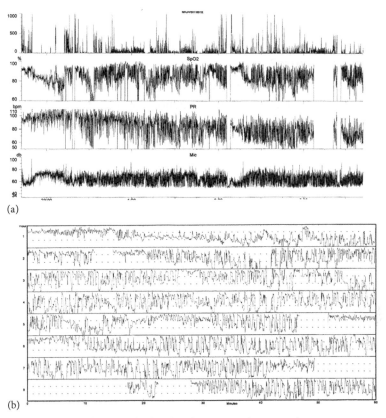

(a)

(b)

Fig. 12.2 (a) A visilab sleep study showing from top to bottom—frequent movements, recurrent SaO_2 desaturation, pulse rate variability and loud snoring sound. (b) Eight hours of oximetry recording during sleep showing frequent deep SaO_2 desaturation dips and period of persistent low SaO_2.

Questions

1 What are the clinical features of acute hypercapnic respiratory failure?

2 What are the common causes of acute hypercapnic respiratory failure?

3 How does obesity affect the respiratory system?

4 What is obesity hypoventilation syndrome, or Pickwickian syndrome?

5 How does OSA/obesity hypoventilation syndrome increase the risk of acute hypercapnic respiratory failure (AHRF)?

in obese patients. Many patients awaiting bariatric surgery report exertional dyspnoea. The load on the ventilatory pump increases due to anterior chest wall encasement with adipose tissue, and the pump becomes weaker due to fatty infiltration of the respiratory muscles. Furthermore, obese patients are more prone to developing respiratory problems, such as basal atelectasis, respiratory infections and hypoxia due to visceral abdominal obesity, particularly when confined to bed over prolonged periods because of impaired diaphragmatic movements, and ventilation at the lung bases and ventilation perfusion abnormalities.

4. What is obesity hypoventilation syndrome, or Pickwickian syndrome?

A few obese patients, usually those who are morbidly obese, have periods of profound hypoventilation during sleep and develop daytime hypercapnia ($pCO_2 > 6$ kPa). The combination of a BMI of >30 and daytime hypercapnia reflecting nocturnal hypoventilation due to obesity in the absence of known causes of respiratory failure is diagnosed as obesity hypoventilation syndrome—previously known as Pickwickian syndrome. Most are morbidly obese and have severe OSA. Nocturnal hypoventilation is indicated by profound hypoxia during sleep with TST below SaO_2 90% >30%, low mean SaO_2 or episodes of prolonged desaturation—$SaO_2 < 88\%$ for 5 minutes.

5. How does OSA/obesity hypoventilation syndrome increase the risk of AHRF?

Patients with undiagnosed OSA associated with hypoventilation are at risk of developing acute ventilatory failure. This may be triggered by an episode of lower respiratory tract infection, bronchospasm or heart failure. Excessive alcohol and benzodiazepine use can also precipitate acute ventilatory failure. This often results in acute admission due to unexplained acute hypercapnic respiratory failure. Many of these patients are admitted to the ITU for mechanical ventilation, resulting in a prolonged hospital stay and an increased risk of mortality. They often have multiple admissions to hospital due to respiratory illness. Early detection of OSA/obesity hypoventilation syndrome and treatment with CPAP can prevent multiple acute admissions with AHRF. Similarly, avoidance of alcohol and benzodiazepine, and prompt treatment of respiratory tract infections in patients known to have OSA/obesity hypoventilation syndrome, can prevent episodes of acute AHRF.

Learning points

Acute hypercapnic/ventilatory respiratory failure is a common condition and may present with drowsiness, reduced level of consciousness and coma without any respiratory symptoms/distress.

Obesity increases the demand on the ventilatory pump and can also weaken the pump causing ventilatory failure—known as obesity hypoventilation syndrome/Pickwickian syndrome.

Most (>90%) patients with obesity hypoventilation syndrome (OHS) have OSA.

OHS should be considered as a cause of acute ventilatory failure, particularly in morbidly obese patients with no known respiratory cause.

Early diagnosis and treatment of obesity hypoventilation prevents morbidity and mortality associated with ventilatory failure.

Further reading

Chakrabarti B, Calverley PM. Management of acute ventilatory failure. Postgrad Med J 2006 Jul;82(969):438–45.

Piper AJ, Grunstein RR. Obesity hypoventilation syndrome: mechanisms and management. Am J Respir Crit Care Med 2011 Feb 1;183(3):292–8.

Sampol G, Rodés G, Ríos J, Romero O, Lloberes P, Morell F. Acute hypercapnic respiratory failure in patients with sleep apneas. Arch Bronconeumol 2010 Sep;46(9):466–72.

A diagnosis of the overlap syndrome was made. His obstructive lung disease was diagnosed as COPD. He was advised regarding smoking cessation and was prescribed appropriate inhaled therapy.

He was referred for non-invasive ventilation and was titrated to pressures of Inspiratory Positive Airway Pressure (IPAP) with 34 cm of water and Expiratory Positive Airway Pressure (EPAP) with 10 cm of water with 1.5 litres of oxygen entrained overnight. With this therapy, his hypoventilation was treated (mean SpO_2 92%) and daytime blood gases significantly improved (pH 7.38, pO_2 12.3 kPa, pCO_2 6.84 kPa).

When he was seen back at the clinic, he felt much better and was less sleepy. After two months on therapy, he was not experiencing any sleepiness at work and his work performance was deemed to be satisfactory. He was discharged from occupational health follow-up.

Questions

1 What is overlap syndrome?
2 When should overlap syndrome be suspected?
3 How is overlap syndrome treated?

Learning points

Patients with overlap syndrome (combination of OSA with COPD) are more symptomatic and at higher risk of pulmonary hypertension and respiratory failure than those with OSA alone.

Patients with overlap syndrome may need overnight oxygen in addition to CPAP.

Further reading

Marin JM et al. Outcomes in patients with chronic obstructive pulmonary disease and sleep apnoea: the overlap syndrome. Am J Respir Crit Care Med 2010;182(3):325–31.
Owens RL et al. Sleep disordered breathing and COPD: the overlap syndrome. Respir Care 2010;55(10):1333–44.

Case 14
Neuropsychological impairment in a psychoanalyst with post-polio syndrome

A 66-year-old man, a non-smoker and wheelchair bound due to post-polio quadriparesis associated with kyphoscoliosis, was referred to the chest clinic for the management of a persistent cough associated with watery sputum of one-year duration. He had poliomyelitis in the 1950s affecting him at cervical cord level. Despite his functional disability due to quadriparesis, he remained active and in good health most of his life, working as a psychoanalyst, except for an episode of type 2 respiratory failure 20 years ago during a post-operative period following haemorrhoid surgery when he required ventilation for a few days. A sleep study at that stage showed no evidence of OSA or nocturnal hypoxia.

He had crackles at the left lung base with dullness on percussion of his chest. His chest X-ray showed scoliosis with volume loss at the right lung base, and a CT scan of the chest showed bronchiectasis with mild dilatation of bronchi in both lower lobes with a distorted lung shape due to quadriparesis. His lung function test showed marked pulmonary restriction with FEV_1 1 litre (32% of predicted) and FVC of 1.1 (28% of predicted). However, his resting oxygen saturations were normal at 96%. He was advised to undergo postural drainage for bronchiectasis.

He also reported worsening oedema of his feet and ankles, despite being on diuretics, and headaches, particularly worse in the early morning. He was suspected to have nocturnal ventilatory problems and an overnight oximetry sleep study was performed (Figure 14.1). This showed marked nocturnal hypoxemia with mean SaO_2 of 85.95% and TST spent below oxygen saturations of 88% (TST<88%) for 5 hours and

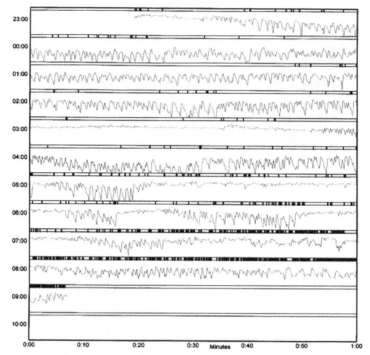

Fig. 14.1 Overnight oximetry study showing repetitive oxygen desaturation pattern of OSA, prolonged period of SaO_2 of desaturation of hypoventilation.

10 minutes (55% of sleep duration). The oximetry pattern showed repeated oxygen desaturations with a 4% oxygen desaturation dip rate of 63.35/hour and prolonged periods of low oxygen saturations.

Review in the sleep clinic revealed that his sleep quality was extremely poor and, on most nights, he had only four hours of interrupted sleep. His sleep was disturbed because of a dry throat and headaches waking him up from sleep. His family members reported loud snoring and obstructed breathing, which was distressing for them to watch. He experienced marked daytime sleepiness which had worsened over the last year, and he could fall asleep in the middle of a conversation. His ESS score was high at 16/24.

He was commenced on CPAP with a nasal mask at fixed pressure of 9 cm of water. However, he could not tolerate the 'brutality' of the CPAP machine, which literally took his 'breath away', and returned it.

He remained symptomatic with markedly disturbed sleep and daytime tiredness. Attempts to adjust the CPAP pressure and CPAP mask were unsuccessful in improving his CPAP tolerance. He was commenced on BiPAP, which he was able to tolerate well, and he noticed an impressive improvement in sleep quality and daytime sleepiness, and a reduction in ankle swelling.

Questions

1 What is post-polio syndrome?
2 Describe the respiratory problems in patients with post-polio syndrome.
3 How do you differentiate between nocturnal hypoventilation and sleep apnoea as a cause of sleep disturbance in post-polio syndrome and does it affect management?

Answers

1. What is post-polio syndrome?

A high proportion (75%) of patients who had polio during child-hood, particularly requiring iron lung ventilation, develop further muscle weakness and fatigue after a latent period of 30 years due to a gradual deterioration of anterior horn cells (motor neurons) in the spinal cord. Further muscle weakness of the respiratory muscles often causes a respiratory problem.

2. Describe the respiratory problems in patients with post-polio syndrome.

The weakness of the abdominal wall muscles (expiratory muscles) reduces the cough effort and sputum clearance and causes retention of sputum. This tends to prolong episodes of respiratory tract infec-tions and make the patients more prone to bronchiectasis. Spinal muscle weakness causes/worsens kyphoscoliosis and further im-pairment of lung function.

The weakness of the inspiratory muscles—diaphragm and inter-costal muscles—causes a reduction in vital capacity. During sleep, there is a further reduction in vital capacity due to the supine body position, reduction in the ventilatory drive and loss of extra dia-phragmatic respiratory muscle tone during REM sleep. These ven-tilatory changes during sleep cause nocturnal hypoventilation. Patients with reduced vital capacity (<50%) are at risk of nocturnal hypoventilation. They may present with disturbed sleep, insomnia, anxiety about going to sleep, inability to breathe on lying flat (ortho-pnoea), choking episodes during sleep, night sweats, early morning headaches, daytime tiredness, and impaired memory and reduced concentration. Nocturnal hypoventilation is suggested by episodes of prolonged oxygen desaturations—SaO_2 for less than 88% for five minutes on an overnight oximetry sleep study. Weakness of the pha-ryngeal muscles and residual effect of poliomyelitis on the brainstem respiratory centre makes them prone to sleep apnoea. The apnoea can be both obstructive and central, and is mainly seen during NREM. Recurrent episodes of apnoeas during sleep cause repetitive oxygen desaturation, disturbed sleep and daytime sleepiness. They rarely report breathlessness during the daytime because of reduced mobility and daytime resting SaO_2 are normal. However, with a further increase in the weakness of respiratory muscles and a reduction in vital capacity, they develop daytime ventilatory failure and hypoxia.

3. How do you differentiate between nocturnal hypoventilation and sleep apnoea as a cause of sleep disturbance in post-polio syndrome and does it affect management?

Obstructive sleep apnoea causes a repetitive sawtooth pattern of desaturation compared to episodes of prolonged oxygen desaturation <88% lasting for five minutes or more due to nocturnal hypoventilation. It is important to establish the relative contribution of sleep apnoea and nocturnal hypoventilation to sleep disturbance and daytime symptoms in patients with post-polio syndrome to decide if they should be treated with CPAP or BiPAP. OSA patients who have reduced vital capacity of <50% are likely to have significant associated hypoventilation, and are less likely to respond to CPAP and to require BiPAP.

Detailed assessment of 35 patients with post-polio syndrome with sleep studies and arterial blood gases showed that more than 50% had OSA, and others had hypoventilation or a combination of hypoventilation with OSA. The latent period after onset of polio was 37 years before the problems described here were noted. Daytime sleepiness was a common symptom in these patients. Patients who had scoliosis or restricted lung function tests were more likely to have hypoventilation.

Learning points

Patients with a history of childhood poliomyelitis are at risk of developing post-polio syndrome after a latent period of 30 to 40 years.

Post-polio syndrome patients are at risk of developing respiratory problems due to the worsening of respiratory muscles weakness.

Disturbed sleep and daytime sleepiness in post-polio syndrome could be due to OSA, nocturnal hypoventilation or a combination of the two.

OSA is mainly due to weakness of the upper airway muscles and responds well to CPAP.

Reduced vital capacity due to respiratory muscle weakness and kyphoscoliosis is the main cause of nocturnal hypoventilation, which can progress to diurnal hypoventilation and respiratory failure. This usually requires nocturnal BiPAP.

Further reading

Dean AC, Graham BA, Dalakas M, Sato S. Sleep apnea in patients with postpolio syndrome. Ann Neurol 1998 May;43(5):661–4.

Howard RS. Poliomyelitis and the postpolio syndrome. BMJ 2005 Jun 4;330(7503):1314–18. Review.

Hsu AA, Staats BA. 'Postpolio' sequelae and sleep-related disordered breathing. Mayo Clin Proc 1998 Mar;73(3):216–24.

Case 15
Nocturnal choking in a patient with a goitre and retrosternal extension

A 70-year-old man with a long-standing goitre and retrosternal extension was referred to a sleep clinic by an endocrinologist. The patient's wife reported that he snored very loudly and was audible even outside the bedroom, and she was worried about his frequent pauses in breathing and choking episodes. However, he slept well without any sleep disturbance. He woke up unrefreshed in the morning and felt sleepy during the daytime, but scored only 2/24 on the ESS. He was retired, smoked 30 cigarettes a day and drank four bottles of wine per week. He was obese, weighing 100 kg for his height of 176 cm with a BMI of 32.2. He had a visible goitre and his neck size at the cricoid cartilage was 47 cm. His oral cavity was narrow, with a Mallampati score of 4. Flow volume loop studies showed mild flattening of the inspiratory and expiratory loops and no sawtooth pattern on the expiratory flow loop. The Empey Index—ratio of FEV1 (ml/s) and PEFR (l/min)—was normal at 6.4 (normal <8–10), but the maximal expiratory flow at 50% FVC (MEF50)/maximal inspiratory flow at 50% FVC (MIF50) was raised at 1.66 (normal <0.8) (Figure 15.1). The CT scan of the neck showed a large goitre with retrosternal extension causing tracheal compression, narrowing and displacement (Figure 15.2). A sleep study confirmed severe OSA—AHI of 51.4 and SaO_2 dip rate of 68.3/hour and mean SaO_2 of 88.8%. The AHI consisted of 44% apnoea and 56% hypopnoea. The apnoeas were obstructive, with the longest apnoea lasting for 49.5 seconds and the mean duration of apnoeas was 17.4 seconds. The patient

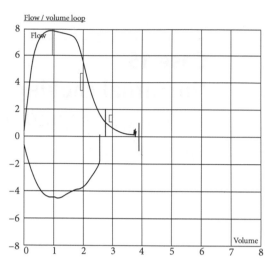

Fig. 15.1 Flow volume showing some flattening of inspiratory and expiratory loop with raised MEF50/MIF50 at 1.66 (normal <0.8) with normal Empey Index indicating floppy pharynx and absence of significant tracheal obstruction.

received a trial of CPAP. His wife reported that he stopped snoring and did not have apnoeas during sleep. He noticed an improvement in his breathing during sleep, but was unable to use CPAP on a regular basis because of psychological barrier—he did not like using CPAP! He had debulking surgery of the neck goitre and retrosternal extension. His snoring and witnessed apnoea subsided and a repeat sleep study showed a reduction in his AHI to 14.6.

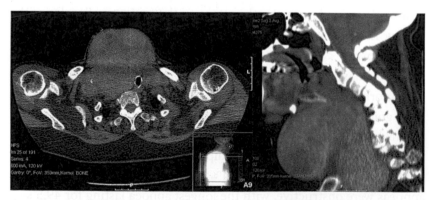

Fig. 15.2 CT scan of neck showing large goitre with retrosternal causing tracheal narrowing and displacement.

Questions

1 How does the spirometry flow volume loop help with diagnosis of upper airway obstruction?

2 Do thyroid problems cause or contribute to upper airway obstruction in OSA?

3 Are cigarette smoking and drinking alcohol risk factors for OSA?

Answers

1. How does the spirometry flow volume loop help with diagnosis of upper airway obstruction?

The flow volume loop can differentiate fixed upper airway obstruction due to tracheal compression from goitre from variable upper airway obstruction at the pharyngeal level in OSA. The maximum inspiratory flow volume (MIFV) is greatly reduced at the mid-lung volume compared to the maximum expiratory flow volume (MEFV) in patients with floppy upper airways. This results in maximal expiratory flow at 50% FVC (MEF50)/maximal inspiratory flow at 50% FVC (MIF50) ratio of >1.0 (normal <0.8), and the MIFV curve has a characteristic truncated shape. In patients with fixed extra-thoracic airway obstruction, the MEFV curve will also show truncation of flows, especially peak expiratory flow, and the MEF50/MIF50 is normal and Empey Index is high.

Furthermore, a sawtooth pattern on the expiratory loop of flow volume also indicates variable upper airway obstruction due to narrow and floppy airways, and supports the diagnosis of OSA (Figure 15.3). It is highly specific, though not seen so often (low

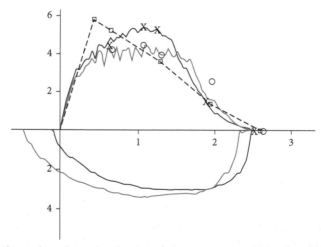

Fig. 15.3 Flow volume loop showing sawtooth pattern on expiratory loop, high MEF50/MIF50 ratio and truncated inspiratory flow volume loop in an obese OSA patient with a big neck.

sensitivity) in patients with OSA. Therefore, an incidental finding of a sawtooth pattern on the spirometry flow volume loop should prompt a diagnosis of OSA.

2. Do thyroid problems cause or contribute to upper airway obstruction in OSA?

Patients with a large goitre are at risk of OSA. The exact mechanisms are not known, but OSA is mainly seen in patients with very large goitres associated with tracheal narrowing or retrosternal extension. Venous obstruction due to retrosternal goitre may cause upper airway congestion and swelling, and a large goitre could interfere with upper airway muscle activity/action.

Patients with hypothyroidism are at an increased risk of OSA. They have a high prevalence (>25%) of OSA. Excessive deposition of mucopolysaccharides soft tissue around the pharynx and tongue (macroglossia) causes upper airway narrowing in patients with untreated hypothyroidism. Similarly, a reduced upper airway muscle tone due to hypotonia contributes to upper airway narrowing and collapsibility. Thyroxine replacement cures OSA in such patients.

3. Are cigarette smoking and drinking alcohol risk factors for OSA?

Cigarette smoking increases the risk of OSA through its effect on upper air inflammation. The inflamed upper airways are narrow and more collapsible. It is known that a current smoker has a higher prevalence of snoring and sleep apnoea than an ex- or non-smoker (Figure 15.4). Smoking-related small airway disease can worsen the effect of apnoeas on oxygen desaturation. Finally, COPD due to smoking increases the risk of ventilatory/respiratory failure in OSA (overlap syndrome).

Alcohol has been shown to precipitate OSA in snorers and worsen sleep apnoea, and increase the duration and severity of apnoeas and hypoxia in patients with OSA. The effect of alcohol on sleep apnoea is marked during the first hour of sleep after alcohol intake. This is mainly due to alcohol-induced hypotonia and respiratory depression. Alcohol-induced diuresis and nocturia may further contribute

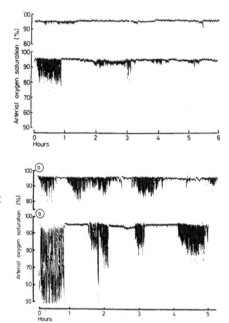

Fig. 15.4 Oximetry sleep studies without and with alcohol in (a) snorers and (b) sleep apnoea patients demonstrating alcohol intake inducing sleep apnoea in snorers and worsening sleep apnoea. **Source:** Reproduced from Journal of Neurology, Neurosurgery and Psychiatry, F G Issa, C E Sullivan, 45, 353–359, © 1982 with permission from BMJ Publishing Group Ltd.

to sleep disturbance in sleep apnoea. Epidemiological studies have shown a variable association between self-reported alcohol consumption and sleep apnoea, particularly in men. Nevertheless, OSA patients should avoid alcohol before bedtime.

Learning points

Presence of sawtooth pattern on expiratory limb of flow volume loop and an increase in MEF50/MIF50 should be investigated for OSA.

A large goitre with retrosternal extension can cause OSA.

Cigarette smoking and alcohol intake increase the risk of OSA.

Further reading

Deegan PC, McNamara VM, Morgan WE. Goitre: a cause of obstructive sleep apnoea in euthyroid patients. Eur Respir J 1997 Feb;10(2):500–2.

Issa FG, Sullivan CE. Alcohol, snoring and sleep apnoea. J Neurol Neurosur Ps 1982;45:353–9.

Shore ET, Millman RF. Abnormalities in the flow-volume loop in obstructive sleep apnoea sitting and supine. Thorax 1984;39:775–9.

Case 16
OSA persists despite removal of a pituitary tumour causing acromegaly

A 65-year-old man with acromegaly was confirmed to have severe OSA when he presented with lethargy and sleepiness, and was treated with CPAP. He was compliant with CPAP and slept well, and did not have EDS (ESS score 5/24). He weighed 89.9 kg for his height of 165 cm (BMI 33) and his collar size was 40.2 cm. He had a transsphenoidal removal of pituitary macro adenoma six months later. He felt better with an improvement in the size of his hands, but he has some impairment of his sense of smell and taste after surgery. He also noticed that his hair was turning darker in colour. A repeat sleep study after pituitary surgery showed persistent sleep apnoea and he remained on CPAP.

Questions

1 How common is sleep apnoea in acromegaly patients?

2 What is the cause of OSA in acromegaly?

3 Does cure of acromegaly improve or eliminate sleep apnoea?

4 Is it safe to use CPAP after transsphenoidal surgery?

Answers

1. How common is sleep apnoea in acromegaly patients?

Most patients with acromegaly have some degree of OSA. The prevalence varies from 27–100%—it tends to be more common in acromegaly patients with an active disease and elevated GH/IGF1 (growth hormone and insulin-like growth factor) levels than patients in remission. OSA is one of the main causes of fatigue and reduced quality of life in acromegaly. It increases the cardiovascular risk associated with acromegaly. Upper airway oedema due to transsphenoidal surgery in acromegaly patients with OSA can increase the risk of post-operative respiratory problems. Screening sleep study is advisable in all patients with acromegaly. Diagnosis and treatment of OSA with CPAP prior to pituitary surgery is likely to reduce peri-operative complications.

2. What is the cause of OSA in acromegaly?

OSA in acromegaly is due to excessive soft tissue deposition of glycosaminoglycan causing a large tongue, hypertrophy of pharyngeal tissue (soft palate) and mucosal thickening of the upper airway. Associated craniofacial abnormalities, such as a protruding jaw, can cause upper airway narrowing—on jaw opening, the tongue base is driven back and narrows the upper airway. Some acromegaly patients are obese and have hypothyroidism contributing to OSA.

3. Does cure of acromegaly improve or eliminate sleep apnoea?

Treatment of acromegaly (surgical or medical) may lead to complete reversal of OSA, but in a substantial proportion (40%) of patients it persists. Excessive soft tissue deposition may regress after treatment of acromegaly (Figure 16.1), but the bony abnormalities persist. Similarly persistent obesity in some patients could account for lack of improvement in OSA after the surgery. Therefore, OSA patients should be re-evaluated after treatment of acromegaly. OSA is more likely to persist in obese acromegaly patients.

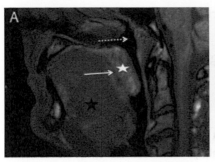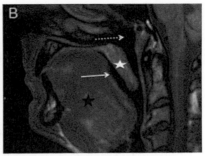

Fig. 16.1 Sagittal T1-weighted MRI sequences of the neck before (a) and after (b) effective treatment of acromegaly in a male patient with OSA. The treatment of acromegaly allowed a clear decrease in thickness of the tongue (*black star*), soft palate (*white star*) and pharyngeal walls, and an opening of the oropharynx space (*solid arrow*) between the tongue and soft palate and of the posterior nasopharynx area (*dashed arrow*), which were associated with the cure of OSA in this patient.
Source: Reproduced from The Journal of Clinical Endocrinology & Metabolism, Pierre Attal, and Philippe Chanson, 'Endocrine Aspects of Obstructive Sleep Apnea', 95:2, pp. 483–495, Copyright 2010, The Endocrine Society.

4. Is it safe to use CPAP after transsphenoidal surgery?

Following most surgical procedures under general anaesthesia, it is recommended that patients should be on CPAP soon after the surgery to prevent post-operative hypoxia due to apnoeic episodes. However, patients on CPAP following transsphenoidal surgery carries a risk of introducing air into the cranium (pneumocephalus), and is therefore contraindicated for at least three to six weeks. This also applies to patients who had upper airway/head and neck surgery where positive upper airways pressure carries a risk of introducing air into the cavities, such as the middle ear, or causing tissue disruption. Measures such as reduction in the post-operative use of opioid/sedation, nursing patients in a propped-up/upright position, supplementary oxygen, and keeping upper airways open with a mandibular advancement splint and nasal airway tube can prevent post-operative hypoxia until it is safe to use CPAP.

Learning points

Obstructive sleep apnoea is very common in patients with acromegaly and contributes to morbidity due to acromegaly.

OSA improves with treatment of acromegaly in some patients, but may persist in others.

CPAP should not be used following transsphenoidal surgery due to the risk of pneumocephalus.

Further reading

Davi' MV, Dalle Carbonare L, Giustina A, Ferrari M, Frigo A, Lo Cascio V, Francia G. Sleep apnoea syndrome is highly prevalent in acromegaly and only partially reversible after biochemical control of the disease. Eur J Endocrinol 2008 Nov;159(5):533–40.

Kopelovich JC, de la Garza GO, Greenlee JD, Graham SM, Udeh CI, O'Brien EK. Pneumocephalus with BiPAP use after transsphenoidal surgery. J Clin Anesth 2012 Aug;24(5):415–18.

Case 17
CPAP transformed my life

A 39-year-old bus driver was referred to a sleep clinic by her GP. She complained of sleepiness—usually while watching television, but more recently she was increasingly sleepy at the cinema. She did not have a regular bed partner, but her children heard her snore. She rated her ESS score at 12/24. She had a past medical history of anaemia, but otherwise was in good health. She worked as a bus driver and held a public service vehicle (PSV) driving licence. She denied ever having fallen asleep at the wheel of the bus. She was obese, with a BMI of 42, but examination otherwise was unremarkable. Her sleep study confirmed severe sleep apnoea (4% dip rate 40 events/hour, minimum SpO_2 66%). She was commenced on CPAP at a fixed pressure of 12 cm of water via a nasal CPAP mask. CPAP compliance check with auto-titrating CPAP showed excellent compliance (Figure 17.1).

At review in clinic, she said that she had never felt better. She had gone to the cinema with her daughter and, for the first time in ten years, she was able to stay awake right through the film. Her daughter no longer reported any snoring. Her ESS was now 6/24. In retrospect, she felt that she might have had sleep apnoea for ten years or more before seeking medical attention.

She informed the diving vehicle licensing agency (DVLA) of her diagnosis and, with the support of her employer, was re-deployed to a desk job until she was established on CPAP. She was reviewed in the clinic after she was established on CPAP and a medical report was sent to the DVLA. Her PSV licence was renewed and she remains under clinic review while she holds a PSV licence.

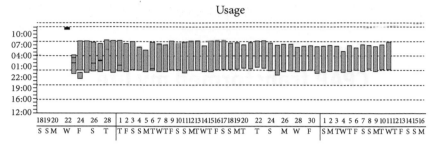

Fig. 17.1 Showing CPAP compliance check—patient used CPAP every night.

Questions

1 What is the lag time for the diagnosis of sleep apnoea?

2 What opportunities are there for screening patients for sleep apnoea?

3 What are the consequences of untreated sleep apnoea?

Answers

1. What is the lag time for the diagnosis of sleep apnoea?

Patients who are diagnosed with sleep apnoea, often in retrospect, have had symptoms for many years (>10 years) before they come to medical attention and diagnosis. This is likely to occur for a variety of reasons. Patients are often unaware of their symptoms and may become habituated to sleepiness so that they no longer perceive it. It often takes concerns from a bed partner before medical assistance is sought.

During medical training, very little sleep medicine is taught within the curriculum. A recent survey of medical undergraduate teaching in the UK found that the median teaching for all aspects of sleep medicine (pathology, pharmacology and diagnostic evaluation) was 2.5 hours. Of the medical schools that responded to the survey, 13% had no teaching whatsoever in their syllabus. Similarly, there is little postgraduate teaching on sleep within the UK. It is therefore perhaps unsurprising that medical professionals themselves may have difficulties in recognizing the signs and symptoms of sleep apnoea. Even when patients present with clinical features of sleep apnoea, there may be poor recognition by the medical profession.

2. What opportunities are there for screening patients for sleep apnoea?

There are numerous opportunities for recognizing patients with un-diagnosed sleep apnoea. Research suggests that, in the ten years prior to OSA diagnosis, patients with OSA made almost twice as many visits to healthcare professionals than age, gender and geographically matched controls. Thus, it seems that patients with OSA have more contact with health professionals than those without, providing opportunity for physicians and other professionals to recognize this common condition.

It is known that untreated OSA leads to an increase in hypertension and treating OSA with CPAP can reduce hypertension. Thus, both primary care and secondary physicians treating patients with hypertension who require more than two drugs for its treatment should specifically ask about symptoms of OSA and refer them to a sleep clinic if required.

Finally, there is a high prevalence of sleep apnoea in patients with type 2 diabetes mellitus. Often symptoms of OSA, such as sleepiness and nocturia, may be attributed to type 2 diabetes mellitus. However, this group of patients should be specifically asked about OSA symptoms. They are often reviewed annually by their GP or at a diabetic clinic, providing opportunities for referral for sleep investigations.

3. What are the consequences of untreated sleep apnoea?

Patients with untreated sleep apnoea may present with un-refreshing sleep, daytime sleepiness and an inability to maintain normal daytime alertness. They may experience difficulties at work due to sleepiness and are at increased risk of motor vehicle accidents and industrial accidents.

Patients may also experience frequent nocturia. This is probably related to atrial dilatation occurring during apnoeas with resultant increased secretion of atrial naturetic peptide, although its presence is often attributed to other common comorbidities, such as diabetes.

Untreated sleep apnoea is associated with hypertension. This is mainly related to an increase in blood pressure during recurrent OSA. Thus, patients, especially those who require more than one anti-hypertensive agent, should be questioned about symptoms of sleep apnoea.

Patients with undiagnosed sleep apnoea may have significant issues after general anaesthesia due to loss of the usual arousal mechanisms as well as post-operative changes in lung physiology. While the effects are likely to depend on the site of surgery and the type of anaesthetic being used, current recommendations suggest that anaesthetists seeing patients at pre-assessment clinics should question relevant patients about symptoms of sleep apnoea. In addition, there may be a correlation between patients who are difficult to intubate and previously unrecognized sleep apnoea. This may be related to a narrow upper airway which may be associated with both scenarios. Anaesthetists may wish to consider referring such patients for formal sleep evaluation.

Learning points

There is a long delay between onset of symptoms of OSA and diagnosis due to lack of awareness among the population and insufficient education in health professionals.

Undiagnosed and untreated OSA can lead to poor quality of life, reduced performance at work, driving-related accidents and an increase in cardiovascular risk.

CPAP is the most effective treatment for OSA and leads to resolution of symptoms, an improvement in quality of life, and a reduction in risk of driving-related accidents and cardiovascular morbidity.

Further reading

Ronald J et al. Health care utilisation in the 10 years prior to diagnosis in obstructive sleep apnoea syndrome patients. Sleep 1999;15:225–9.

Urquhart DS et al. Survey of undergraduate sleep medicine teaching in UK medical schools. Arch Dis Child 2012;97:90–1.

Case 18
Persistent daytime sleepiness despite CPAP

A 58-year-old obese man of Indian origin, with a history of coronary artery disease, was suspected to have OSA by the cardiologist because of his symptoms of daytime somnolence and heavy snoring. He was extremely sleepy during the daytime and could nod off watching television, reading a book or sitting in a waiting area and even when talking to people. He frequently slept while travelling on a bus or train. Daytime sleepiness used to affect his work when he worked as a civil servant. He often felt sleepy while driving and reduced his driving to a few miles only for fear of having an accident—he pulled over for a rest when he felt sleepy. He scored 21/24 on the ESS. He snored very loudly and kept his wife awake, and she often slept in a separate room. His sleep was disturbed—he often woke himself up from his own snoring at night. He woke up unrefreshed and tired in the morning. He had put on weight gradually over the last few years. He was mildly obese, with a BMI of 30.91, collar size of 43.3 cm and grade 4 size oral cavity on the Mallampati scoring system. A visilab sleep study (overnight oximetry and audio-visual recording) confirmed OSA, with a SaO_2 dip rate of 32.4 and mean SaO_2 of 94%, and loud snoring up to 80db. The oxygen desaturation pattern was characteristic of OSA. He was titrated with CPAP at a fixed pressure of 9 cm of water via a nasal CPAP mask and a repeat sleep study on CPAP showed complete elimination of OSA—the SaO_2 dip rate was 1.29 and mean SaO_2 were 97.64. His wife noted a significant improvement in his sleep quality and he no longer snored on CPAP. She was also able to have a restful night's sleep. He was less tired, but remained sleepy with an ESS score of 16 despite a good response to CPAP.

He was found to have mild anaemia, which was being investigated. He was very compliant with CPAP and reported using it every night for seven hours, and was happy to persist with treatment. He still felt very somnolent and his ESS score remained high at 21—he often dropped off to sleep sitting down in the evenings. Otherwise, daytime sleepiness did not affect his other daytime activities—he retired from his work and only drove to the local shops. He was not keen on taking the stimulant, modafinil, for his sleepiness.

Questions

1 How common is persistent EDS despite CPAP in OSA?

2 What is the initial management of patients who report persistent daytime sleepiness despite CPAP?

3 What is the next step in patients who have persistent EDS, despite good objective demonstration of good CPAP compliance?

4 Are there any therapeutic options for persistent daytime sleepiness?

Answers

1. How common is persistent EDS despite CPAP in OSA?

Persistent daytime sleepiness despite CPAP is common; studies have found a prevalence of 20–40%. Management requires a careful systematic approach to identify and treat the causes of EDS.

EDS is one of the main presenting symptoms of OSA. The ESS remains the best tool available to assess the severity of EDS and response. An ESS score of <11 is considered normal, 11–14 mild, 15–18 moderate and >18 severe. The treatment of OSA with CPAP reduces the ESS score by an average of 2.9—much higher in patients with moderate to severe OSA than mild OSA.

2. What is the initial management of patients who report persistent daytime sleepiness despite CPAP?

It is important to assess an overall improvement in symptoms of OSA, including the elimination of snoring, improved sleep quality, waking up fresh in the morning and feeling less tired and sleepy during the daytime, rather than purely relying on a reduction in ESS.

It is not uncommon for some patients to report no or little change in ESS, despite an overall improvement in OSA symptoms. OSA patients have a high prevalence of depression and report tiredness and fatigue. It is important that fatigue and tiredness due to depression is not misinterpreted as daytime sleepiness.

Suboptimal compliance with CPAP is one of the common causes of persistent symptoms including daytime sleepiness. It has been shown that OSA patients need to use CPAP for at least four hours every night to notice an improvement in daytime sleepiness. Longer hours of CPAP use results in further improvement in daytime sleepiness—the more, the better. Missing CPAP even for a single night can lead to a rapid return of symptoms.

An improvement in OSA symptoms with CPAP is rapid, even after the first night's use—patients may report waking up fresh and not sleepy. However, it may take up to four weeks for the maximum response and, in a few, it may be delayed up to three months. In some patients, a lack of immediate improvement in the symptoms with a burden of using CPAP affects compliance. An objective CPAP compliance may demonstrate suboptimal compliance as a cause of persistent daytime sleepiness. The compliance check may also detect air leakage from the nasal CPAP mask as a cause of reduced effectiveness. Air leakage due to a poor fitting CPAP mask, or mouth breathing that is noisy and uncomfortable, can further reduce CPAP compliance. However, some OSA patients remain excessively sleepy, despite good compliance with CPAP.

3. What is the next step in patients who have persistent EDS, despite good objective demonstration of good CPAP compliance?

Persistent symptoms despite good CPAP compliance may be due to an insufficient fixed CPAP pressure. It is known that sleep apnoea varies in severity during the night in different body positions and sleep stages, and from night to night. A fixed CPAP pressure set based on a CPAP titration sleep study may not be sufficient to abolish OSA every night. A repeat sleep study on CPAP may help to detect persistent sleep apnoea on a fixed CPAP pressure. However, a single night sleep study may miss night-to-night variation in the sleep apnoea severity. A pragmatic approach may be to increase the CPAP pressure or use an auto-titrating CPAP. An auto-CPAP machine detects apnoea and varies the pressure required to eliminate apnoea.

In others, the lack of effectiveness of CPAP in improving daytime sleepiness may be due to co-existing conditions causing daytime sleepiness. OSA diagnosed on oximetry cannot distinguish between OSA and CSA as a cause of recurrent oxygen desaturations. In patients with mixed apnoeas, CPAP unmasks central apnoea—complex sleep apnoea. This can be detected with the help of a multichannel sleep study that includes respiratory monitoring during sleep. Patients with complex sleep apnoea have persistent apnoea and daytime sleepiness despite CPAP, and often require BiPAP.

A few patients with OSA have associated neurological conditions, such as periodic limb movement syndrome (PLMS), as a cause of disturbed sleep and daytime sleepiness. OSA has been implicated as a cause of PLMS. A detailed PSG often helps to identify these coexisting causes of EDS.

EDS is a common feature of hypothalamic disorders (syndrome) (Table 18.1). These patients may have associated obesity due to hypothalamic dysfunction as a cause of OSA. Correction of OSA with CPAP will only eliminate OSA-related daytime sleepiness and have no effect on hypersomnia due to underlying hypothalamic disorders.

Nevertheless, a few OSA patients may develop neuroanatomical and neurofunctional changes as a result of long-standing undiagnosed OSA, which may account for the lack of improvement in sleep quality or daytime sleepiness.

Table 18.1 Potential causes of EDS in adults

- fragmented sleep (quality of sleep)
- sleep deprivation (quantity of sleep)
- shift work
- depression
- narcolepsy
- hypothyroidism
- restless leg syndrome/periodic limb movement disorder
  - drugs
  - sedatives
  - stimulants (caffeine, theophyllines, amphetamines)
  - β-blockers
- selective serotonin reuptake inhibitors (SSRIs)
- idiopathic hypersomnolence
- excess alcohol
- neurological conditions
  - dystrophia myotonica
  - previous encephalitis
  - previous head injury
  - parkinsonism

Source: Scottish Intercollegiate Guidelines Network (SIGN). Management of Obstructive Sleep Apnoea/Hypopnoea in Adults. Edinburgh: SIGN; 2003. (SIGN publication no. 73).

4. Are there any therapeutic options for persistent daytime sleepiness?

Modafinil is a central nervous system stimulant without the addictive properties of amphetamine, and promotes wakefulness. It can be a useful adjunct to CPAP in a dose of 200–400 mg in CPAP compliant patients with persistent daytime sleepiness (>6 hours/night). It also improves alertness and quality of life. It is generally well tolerated and, if taken before midday, does not affect night-time sleep. Headaches and nausea are the two most common side effects, and it should be used with caution in patients with hypertension and heart disease.

Armodafinil is a long-acting isomer of modafinil with a half-life of 10 to 15 hours, and has also been shown to be effective in improving daytime sleepiness.

Learning points

Persistent daytime sleepiness despite CPAP treatment is common.

Reduced CPAP compliance and effectiveness should be excluded by objective measurement of CPAP compliance and CPAP sleep study respectively before considering further management.

EDS is a common symptom and should be distinguished from fatigue and tiredness.

If EDS is due to depression, the side effects of drugs and metabolics should be considered.

OSA is often associated with neurological disorders such as PLMS and narcolepsy—a PSG should be done to exclude these conditions.

Further reading

Kay GG, Feldman N. Effects of armodafinil on simulated driving and self-report measures in obstructive sleep apnea patients prior to treatment with continuous positive airway pressure. J Clin Sleep Med 2013 May 15;9(5):445–54.

Management of obstructive sleep apnoea/hypopnoea in adults. A national clinical guideline. Scottish Intercollegiate Guidelines Network (SIGN). 2003.

Case 19
CPAP intolerance and non-compliance—treatment with MAS

A 36-year-old male accountant presented with long-standing snoring with a little sleep disturbance and daytime sleepiness five years ago. His sleep study confirmed OSA with an AHI of 25. In view of the asymptomatic nature of his OSA, he was treated with a custom-made MAS. He found the splint to be uncomfortable and ineffective in abolishing his snoring. It broke after a while and he stopped using it. Over the next few years, he gained weight and his snoring worsened. A repeat sleep study showed worsening of OSA with a SaO_2 dip rate of 57.8 and mean SaO_2 of 88.7%. He was treated with CPAP at a fixed pressure of 9 cm of water. His snoring and sleep apnoea completely subsided with the elimination of OSA—the SaO_2 dip rate on CPAP was 0.5/hour with mean SaO_2 of 97.4%. He benefited from CPAP and used it for a year, but did not like the prospect of being on it long term. He also experienced the side effects of persistent nasal blockage, despite nasal steroids, humidification of air and nasal surgery.

He was not obese and did attempt improve his fitness, but this had no effect on his snoring. He was not too keen on using an MAS again because of his past experience and the non-curative nature of the treatment. He was referred to an ENT surgeon who found that he had grade 2 hypertrophy of the tonsils, a lax soft palate, a prominent tongue pushing the epiglottis backward and 75% upper airway collapse at the oropharynx on Muller's manoeuvre. He was arranged to have a sleep nasendoscopy with a plan for two-stage ENT surgery—tonsillectomy followed by laser assisted palatoplasty (LAUP). Meanwhile, he agreed to see a dentist for another attempt at MAS. He was fitted with a custom-made MAS. He was able to tolerate MAS with the elimination of his snoring and an improvement in the dip rate to 15.5/hour. A further adjustment/advancement of the splint led to a reduction in the dip rate to 4.90/hour. He did not want to have surgery.

Questions

1 What are the main reasons for CPAP intolerance and non-compliance?

2 Are there any curative treatments for OSA?

3 What is the role of MAS in the management of OSA?

Answers

1. What are the main reasons for CPAP intolerance and non-compliance?

Though CPAP is the most effective treatment for OSA, it is not an easy treatment for long-term use. Many patients find it difficult to use every night because of the physical side effects or psychological issues. Overall, 60% patients are able to use it long term. However, identification and correction of problems associated with CPAP use can improve CPAP tolerance and compliance (Table 19.1).

CPAP compliance is likely to be much better if the CPAP treatment is explained to the patient and set up by an experienced sleep technician with proper selection of the CPAP mask and titration of the CPAP pressure.

In the past, a CPAP titration sleep study—a sleep study on CPAP in the sleep laboratory monitored by a sleep technician—was done to set the CPAP pressure. However, this is rarely required these days, as CPAP pressure can be estimated from the physical characteristics of patients with one of the available algorithms or just from experience. In general, it may be preferable to commence CPAP at a lower pressure which the patient is able to tolerate, rather than to aim for the ideal/estimated pressure. The introduction of CPAP at a high pressure can lead to an uncomfortable sensation or difficulty in breathing. Auto-titrating CPAP machines are able to adjust the CPAP pressure by detecting apnoeas and eliminate the need for CPAP titration.

Table 19.1 Common reasons for poor CPAP compliance

- CPAP mask—pressure symptoms (nasal bridge sore)
- CPAP mask—displacement and air leak
- CPAP cold room air—vasomotor rhinitis
- CPAP pressure—too high (uncomfortable) or too low (ineffective)
- CPAP mask—claustrophobia
- CPAP mask appearance—cosmetically unacceptable
- Absence of symptoms

A poorly fitting nasal CPAP mask can cause a pressure sore over the nasal bridge and upper lip. This is more likely to occur if the mask head straps are pulled too tight. With an improvement in mask technology—comfort and a self-sealing mechanism—pressure sores are less of a problem now. Use of other types of CPAP masks, such as nasal cushions/pillows or full-face CPAP masks, may help to avoid pressure symptoms.

CPAP mask displacement during sleep can cause air leakage and a gushing noise. This not only disturbs the patient's sleep, but makes it ineffective in delivering set CPAP pressure. It can be managed by securing the CPAP mask firmly with an adjustable CPAP mask and head straps, placing the CPAP machine nearer to the patient to avoid pulling on the CPAP tubing or using longer CPAP tubing.

CPAP prevents upper airway collapse by increasing upper airway pressure. However, to achieve an increase in upper airway pressure with a nasal CPAP mask, the mouth needs to be closed. Mouth breathers, either due to habitual mouth breathing or nasal obstruction, are likely to experience uncomfortable air leakage from the mouth. This can be prevented by using chin straps to keep the mouth closed during sleep, correction of nasal obstruction or using a full face mask covering both the mouth and nose.

One of the other main problems affecting CPAP tolerance is CPAP rhinitis. This is as a result of cold or dry room air causing reflex vasodilation of nasal mucosal (vasomotor rhinitis) causing nasal congestion and blockage. Poor-quality indoor room air (pollutants/irritants/allergen) may exacerbate underlying allergic rhinitis. Ensuring that the room air is warm and clean, or using CPAP machines with an attached/inbuilt humidifier and heating system, can prevent vasomotor rhinitis. Nasal anticholinergic or steroid sprays can provide short-term relief from rhinitis. An ENT review is helpful in patients with persistent nasal congestion and blockage.

However, in a few patients, the reason for CPAP non-compliance is not due to any of these side effects, but due to a psychosocial barrier against CPAP. They find CPAP either cosmetically unacceptable or feel claustrophobic. A careful explanation of the benefits of CPAP use, reassurance and use of a mild anxiolytic/sedative during the first few weeks of CPAP treatment may help. Cognitive Behavioural Therapy (CBT) may help, particularly in patients who feel claustrophobic with a CPAP mask.

In general, symptomatic patients with EDS are more likely to comply with CPAP than patients with few symptoms. However, a clear explanation regarding the long-term health benefits of CPAP may convince asymptomatic patients to comply with CPAP.

2. Are there any curative treatments for OSA?

Weight loss is the only curative treatment for OSA in obese patients. Obstructive sleep apnoea, hypertension, diabetes mellitus and hyperlipidaemia subside in most patients following weight loss in morbidly obese patients with bariatric surgery. However, not all obese patients can or want to have bariatric surgery and the success rate of achieving long-term weight loss with non-surgical treatments, such as (very) low calorie diets and pharmacological treatment, is low. Moreover, many OSA patients are not obese. Treatment options in such patients are relatively limited even though patients often seek a surgical 'cure'. Tracheostomy and uvulopalatopharyngoplasty (UPPP) was a mainstay of treatment for OSA until the early 1980s. Tracheostomy is extremely effective in treating OSA, but is not acceptable to most patients due to the long-term complications and problems. Systemic reviews have shown that the results of UPPP are inconsistent—a significant improvement in sleep apnoea was seen only in a few studies, 62% of patients reported side effects and many regretted having had surgery.

3. What is the role of MAS in the management of OSA?

Bringing the lower jaw forward advances the tongue forward as well, and enlarges the upper airways and reduces the tendency to collapse. Mandibular advancement devices have been increasingly used as an alternative to CPAP in the treatment of OSA. Several randomized controlled trials comparing MASs with CPAP have shown that the splints are effective, though reduction in AHI is less than with CPAP, but preferred over CPAP. There are many different types of mandibular repositioning devices (MRD) for patients who are unable to tolerate CPAP. These devices are either commercially available or custom made by a dentist. They are fixed or adjustable. Commercially available fixed devices have been used for treatment of OSAH, but their effectiveness has not been confirmed in clinical trials. A recent trial showed that commercially available MRD was not effective and had a high failure rate compared to custom-made MRD. There is good evidence for the effectiveness of custom-made adjustable devices—clinical trials have shown a 40–70% reduction in the AHI. Both patient-adjusted and dentist-adjusted MRDs have been used to achieve maximum tolerable protrusion of the mandible. It is likely that a dentist-adjusted MRD will be more effective in reducing AHI, daytime sleepiness and snoring, and have fewer side effects than a patient-adjusted MRD.

We found about half of patients issued with a custom-made adjustable MAS used it regularly. The splint use was dependent on social circumstances as much as physical symptoms in patients with mild sleep apnoea. In more severe cases in patients with daytime symptoms, the splint was preferred to CPAP and compliance was better. Mild discomfort and excess salivation are common side effects during the early stages of use and occurred in about two-thirds of patients, rarely causing non-compliance.

NICE recommends an MAS for the treatment of mild sleep apnoea, but the recommendation on the exact type of device is not yet available.

Learning points

CPAP tolerance and compliance can be improved by careful identification and correction of problems associated with CPAP use.

Weight loss can cure sleep apnoea, but surgical treatments for OSA are either ineffective or unacceptable.

MASs of an adjustable type are a useful alternative to CPAP, particularly in mild OSA.

Further reading

Franklin KA, Anttila H, Axelsson S, Gislason T, Maasilta P, Myhre KI, Rehnqvist N. Effects and side-effects of surgery for snoring and obstructive sleep apnea—a systematic review. Sleep 2009 Jan;32(1):27–36. Review.

Gordon P, Sanders MH. Sleep.7: positive airway pressure therapy for obstructive sleep apnoea/hypopnoea syndrome. Thorax 2005 Jan;60(1):68–75.

Lim J, Lasserson TJ, Fleetham J, Wright J. Oral appliances for obstructive sleep apnoea. Cochrane Database of Systematic Reviews 2006 Jan;25(1):CD004435.

Case 20
Will not use CPAP—ends up with tracheostomy

A 53-year-old obese Greek Cypriot man was diagnosed to have OSA 13 years ago and was recommended treatment with CPAP. He could not tolerate CPAP and remained without any treatment for OSA. He underwent a planned tonsillectomy under general anaesthesia a year later. As a precaution, a pre-operative tracheostomy was performed. However, attempts to close his tracheostomy after surgery resulted in obstructive breathing during sleep and sleep disturbance. He slept very well with open tracheostomy and did not want his tracheostomy to be closed. He has remained on tracheostomy for the last 13 years for OSA. His wife provides tracheostomy care. He had recurrent lower respiratory infections. He was referred to a chest clinic recently because he coughed up fresh blood from the tracheostomy and mouth. He also reported weight loss of 5 kg. He was an ex-smoker of 5 pack year and had stopped smoking 14 years ago. An emergency ENT endoscopy via tracheostomy revealed no abnormality. His chest X-ray was normal. Bronchoscopy examination showed endotracheal mucosal swelling on the posterior tracheal wall due to granulation tissue (Figures 20.1 and 20.2). He has remained on tracheostomy for the last 13 years for OSA.

Questions

1 What are the risks associated with untreated OSA?
2 What are the pros and cons of tracheostomy for the treatment of OSA?

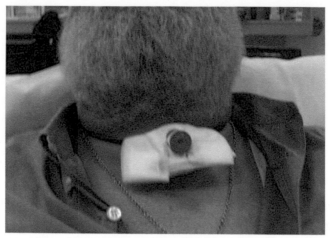

Fig. 20.1 Patient with OSA treated with long-term permanent tracheostomy.

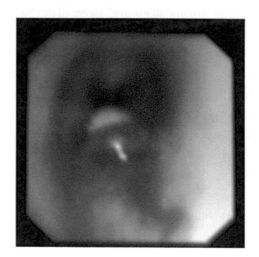

Fig. 20.2 Fibre-optic bronchoscopy view of upper trachea showing red and swollen tracheal mucosa.

Answers

1. What are the risks associated with untreated OSA?

Untreated OSA carries the following risks:

a) *Post-operative complications*: Patients with untreated OSA are at a higher risk of post-operative problems due to the effect of anaesthetic agents and sedatives on the pharyngeal muscle tone, and arousals resulting in airway collapse and depression of ventilation (Table 20.1). The complications are exacerbated by the use of opioids, particularly if given by an intravenous route (PCA) for the control of post-operative pain. Most of the complications are seen during the immediate post-operative period when the patient is likely to be in the recovery room and monitored. However, these complications can occur after a delay of 4 to 12 hours when the patient is likely to be on a ward or discharged (day case) and not under close supervision.

The anaesthetist, aware of the post-operative risks in OSA patients, will substitute general anaesthesia with regional anaesthesia and use NSAIDs instead of opiates for post-operative analgesia. The use of CPAP during the peri-operative period can reduce the post-operative risks in OSA patients. There is evidence that OSA patients well established on CPAP prior to surgery are at a lower risk of post-operative problems.

b) *Cardiovascular risk*: OSA is associated with cardiovascular morbidity due to systemic and pulmonary hypertension, cardiac arrhythmias, coronary artery disease, congestive cardiac failure and stroke. Recent large epidemiological prospective studies and clinical trials have confirmed at least a twofold increased risk of cardiovascular problems and stroke in patients with OSA. The risk is

Table 20.1 Post-operative problems in patients with undiagnosed or untreated OSA

Apnoea, respiratory depression, hypoxia and respiratory arrest
Cardiac arrhythmia and injury
Re-intubation, admission to ITU and longer hospital stay
Unexpected death

closely associated with chronic intermittent hypoxia rather than the AHI. Treatment of OSA with CPAP, particularly in symptomatic/moderate to severe OSA patients, reduces cardiovascular risk.

c) *Road traffic accidents (RTA)*: EDS is thought to be the second most common (20%) cause of RTAs after alcohol. OSA is one of the commonest causes of EDS and neurocognitive impairment and increases the risk of RTAs. Treatment of OSA reduces the risk of driving-related accidents. Patients should be made aware of the risk and their responsibility to inform the DVLA.

d) *Mortality*: An increased risk of death, mainly from cardiovascular causes, was noted among OSA patients when tracheostomy was the only available treatment. The deaths were prevented in patients who accepted tracheostomy for treatment of OSA. Recent large epidemiological studies in patients with OSA, particularly men with severe obstructive apnoea, have shown at least a twofold increase in the risk of death—mainly sudden deaths and cardiovascular deaths. Furthermore, OSA has been linked to death from cancer in a recent American study, showing that patients with severe OSA (AHI >30) had approximately a five times higher chance of dying from cancer.

2. **What are the pros and cons of tracheostomy for the treatment of OSA?**

Tracheostomy was the first treatment for OSA. It was based on the simple concept of bypassing the upper airway obstruction at the supraglottic region. It had one of the most dramatic effects of providing instant relief from OSA with restoration of normal sleep and elimination of daytime sleepiness. Tracheostomy also reduced the mortality rate due to OSA. No deaths occurred in patients treated with tracheostomy, while 10% of patients who were advised to use weight loss as treatment for OSA died of vascular death five years after diagnosis.

However, tracheostomy is associated with long-term problems and complications, such as lower respiratory infections, bleeding and tracheal stenosis. Tracheostomy may have a role in a few selective patients as an interim measure.

Learning points

Untreated OSA increases post-operative problems. Some of these can be serious and life-threatening.

OSA patients have a higher cardiovascular co-morbidity, which adds to the post-operative risk of OSA.

OSA itself at least doubles the risk of cardiovascular disease, particularly in men with severe OSA. The risk appears mainly to be due to chronic intermittent hypoxia.

Similarly, OSA patients have approximately a twofold increase in the risk of death from sudden death, cardiovascular causes and cancer.

CPAP is the most effective treatment for OSA and should be the first choice of treatment, but may be the only option for CPAP-intolerant patients.

Further reading

Adebola O, Adesanya AO, Lee W, Greilich NB, Joshi GP. Perioperative management of obstructive sleep apnea. Chest 2010;138(6):1489–98.

Herder C, Schmeck J, Appelboom DJK, Vries D. Risks of general anaesthesia in people with obstructive sleep apnoea. BMJ 2004;329:955–9.

Case 21
Bariatric surgery cures sleep apnoea

A 39-year-old lady was referred via the bariatric clinic. She lived alone and did not have a regular bed partner. However, when visiting her parents she often had to sleep downstairs, as her snoring disturbed them if she slept on the same floor. She had not noted any particular sleepiness and rated her ESS at 9/21. She did not drive a car. Her past medical history included chronic osteomyelitis for which she eventually required foot amputation, irritable bowel syndrome, non-insulin dependent diabetes mellitus and hypertension. Her regular medications included metformin, losartan, amlodipine and loperamide. Her BMI was 48. Examination was otherwise unremarkable.

She underwent a sleep study which revealed severe sleep apnoea with a 4% dip rate of 113 events/hour. She was commenced on CPAP at 12 cm of water and achieved good compliance. She felt that she had more energy during the day. She did not snore on CPAP and, when visiting her parents, she was able to sleep on the same floor. She subsequently underwent a laparoscopic sleeve gastrectomy. She had an uneventful postoperative recovery and was discharged the next day. She lost 50 kg over four months and her BMI came down to 32. Her diabetes mellitus and hypertension resolved. She found difficulty in using CPAP and was unable to use it for some weeks. Despite not using CPAP, her snoring was no longer audible in other rooms and she did not notice sleepiness or low energy. A repeat sleep study off CPAP showed that her sleep apnoea had resolved with weight loss (4% dip rate 3 events/hour). She returned her machine and was discharged from the clinic.

Questions

1 What are the current guidelines regarding referral of patients for consideration of bariatric surgery?

2 What are the benefits of bariatric surgery?

3 How does weight loss impact on OSA?

Answers

1. What are the current guidelines regarding referral of patients for consideration of bariatric surgery?

Current NICE guidelines suggest that bariatric surgery should be considered in patients with a BMI >40. It should also be considered in patients with a BMI between 35 and 40 who have obesity-associated comorbidity, such as sleep apnoea, hypertension or type 2 diabetes mellitus, which are expected to improve with significant weight loss. There should be evidence that non-surgical methods of weight loss have been attempted for at least six months, but not successful to achieve a sustained weight loss. Patients should be referred to a specialist weight loss service and must be aware that long-term follow-up will be required and they must be willing to comply with this follow-up. However, bariatric surgery should be considered as a first-line option in those with BMI >50, as these patients are unlikely to achieve weight loss through lifestyle changes or drug treatment alone.

2. What are the benefits of bariatric surgery?

Bariatric surgery is a rapidly evolving field and it is likely that indications for bariatric surgery will expand. There is little evidence regarding the current selection criteria for bariatric surgery. Most centres have developed their own selection process, which includes a medical, anaesthetic, dietetic and psychological review to ensure that the patient is physically and psychologically suitable for the surgery. Recommendation for the surgery is usually made at the multi-disciplinary meeting.

The most commonly performed procedures include the Roux en Y gastric bypass (RYGB) and sleeve gastrectomy. Patients with more severe obesity are considered for bilio-pancreatic diversion (BPD). Over 90% of all bariatric surgery is performed laparoscopically.

Mortality for RYGB in expert centres is 0.4%. Early complications include thromboembolism and anastomotic leak, while later complications include cholelithiasis, anastomotic strictures and marginal ulcers. Deficiency of iron, folate, vitamin B12 and fat-soluble vitamins is common and requires long-term supplementation with monitoring of serum levels.

Sleeve gastrectomy has been introduced more recently into mainstream bariatric practice and, thus, there is less long-term data on its use. Complications include haemorrhage, anastomotic leak and stricture at rates which are comparable to RYGB. There is evidence that both operating time and hospital stay are shorter than for RYGB. Long-term nutritional supplementation is required.

While complications of BPD are similar to other procedures, it has traditionally been regarded as a higher risk procedure. However, weight loss is greater than with the other two procedures and there is a higher rate of discontinuation of medical therapy in those with diabetes.

Obese individuals have higher medical costs than the non-obese, primarily due to medication costs for diabetes, hypertension and lipid disorders, and have higher levels of analgesic and psychiatric prescribing. There is also societal loss with individuals having reduced productivity and increased sick leave. These losses can be reversed with bariatric surgery and it is estimated that the costs associated with the surgical intervention are recouped after four years.

3. How does weight loss impact on OSA?

Weight loss following bariatric surgery reduces neck and abdominal obesity and improves upper airway size and functional residual capacity, respectively, which act synergistically to reduce the propensity for upper airway collapse during sleep.

Meta-analysis of large cohorts of bariatric surgical patients has shown resolution of symptoms of OSA in ~85% of patients. However, not all patients have complete resolution of sleep apnoea after bariatric surgery. In a randomized control trial comparing intensive medical intervention to laparoscopic gastric banding (which delivers less weight loss than the procedures outlined here), patients undergoing surgical intervention had greater weight loss at two years than those randomized to medical therapy, but 20% did not have a reduction in AHI in a sleep study after the procedure. This illustrates the multi-factorial aetiology of sleep apnoea, e.g. the effect of upper airway size and neural control. Patients with sleep apnoea should be followed up after bariatric surgery until their weight loss has plateaued. They should then undergo a repeat sleep study to ensure that their sleep apnoea has resolved so that they can stop using CPAP. However, they should be informed prior to surgery that significant weight loss may not entirely ameliorate their sleep apnoea.

Learning points

Bariatric surgery should be considered in morbidly obese OSA patients.

Weight loss following bariatric surgery such as sleeve gastrectomy and gastric bypass not only cures sleep apnoea, but also type 2 diabetes mellitus, hypertension and hyperlipidaemia.

In a few patients, OSA may persist, despite bariatric surgery.

Further reading

Dixon JB, Schachter LM, O'Brien PE et al. Surgical vs conventional therapy for weight loss treatment of obstructive sleep apnoea: A randomised controlled trial. JAMA 2012;308(11):1142–9.

Neff KJH et al. Bariatric surgery: A best practice article. J Clin Pathol 2013;66:90–8.

Padwal R, Klarenbach S, Wiebe N et al. Bariatric surgery: A systematic review of the clinical and economic evidence. J Gen Intern Med 2011;26(10):1183–94.

Case 22
Sleep disturbance and daytime sleepiness persists in a snorer despite CPAP—Periodic Limb Movement Syndrome

A 67-year-old male retired civil engineer was referred to the sleep clinic by an ENT surgeon because of concern that his sleep disturbance may precipitate another heart attack. He had persistent nasal obstruction, despite correction of his deviated nasal septum. His sleep study showed a few oxygen desaturations, and sleep nasendoscopy (midazolam induced sleep) found obstruction at the palatal level with oxygen desaturation to 79%. He had had a recent heart attack and was waiting for a trial of CPAP. He reported having disturbed sleep for at least five years—he woke up from his sleep every five minutes sweating associated with palpitations and a dry throat. He felt extremely tired in the morning and excessively sleepy during the daytime. He invariably slept during train journeys. He snored loudly according to his wife, who also noticed witnessed apnoeas for at least a year. He was of normal body weight (BMI 24.9) and neck size (39 cm), and, despite reported EDS, his ESS score was normal at 8/24. A repeat overnight home oximetry sleep study showed no evidence of OSA. There were no characteristic SaO_2 desaturation dips with a normal SaO_2 dip rate of 3.1/hour and normal mean SaO_2 of 94.3%. He slept well during the sleep study.

He was suspected to have upper airway resistance syndrome (UARS) in view of the history of loud snoring associated with sleep disturbance and daytime sleepiness, but had a normal oximetry sleep study and was given a therapeutic trial of CPAP. He was very compliant with CPAP and used it for more than seven hours every night on objective compliance check. He reported a slight improvement in his sleep quality and daytime sleepiness. He was provided with a custom-made MAS for long-term treatment of UARS, but did not benefit. He reverted to CPAP, but found no improvement. A further overnight oximetry sleep study showed no evidence of OSA.

He remained concerned about his sleep disturbance and presented to a local A&E department because of the inability to breathe and associated palpitations and sweating. He was referred to the neurology sleep specialist and reported that his legs 'jumped' during sleep, and a diagnosis of PLMS was suspected. Polysomnography (PSG) revealed disrupted sleep and reduced sleep efficiency (84%) (Figure 22.1). There were frequent limb movements, mainly affecting the legs, often causing arousal or awakening (Periodic Limb Movement Index 36/hour) (Figure 22.2). In addition to these movements was an occasional loss of REM atonia, with bursts of phasic EMG activity (Figure 22.3). There was no significant sleep-related breathing problem. He responded well to treatment with clonazepam.

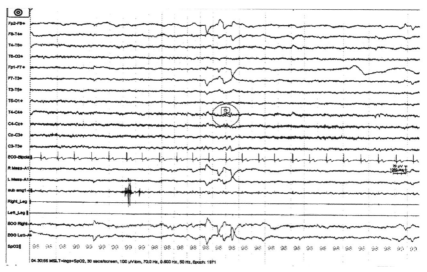

Fig. 22.1 Showing phasic muscle (EMG) activity during REM sleep at 4.30.55.

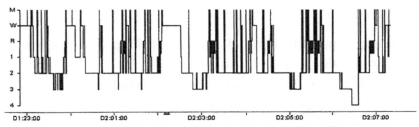

Fig. 22.2 Hypnogram showing disrupted sleep and reduced sleep efficiency.

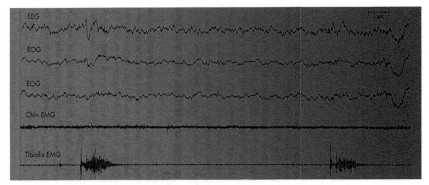

Fig. 22.3 Showing periodic burst of anterior tibialis muscle activity (tibialis EMG) associated with an arousal on EEG.

Source: All I Want Is A Good Night's Sleep: Practical Advice for You and Your Family Sonia Ancoli-Israel PhD (Author) Publication Date: 9 May 1996 | ISBN-10: 0815148437 | ISBN-13: 978-0815148432.

Questions

1 What is the differential diagnosis of sleep disruption and daytime sleepiness in a snorer?

2 What are the common movement disorders during sleep?

3 What is PLMS?

Answers

1. What is the differential diagnosis of sleep disruption and daytime sleepiness in a snorer?

Snoring is extremely common, and sleep disturbance and daytime sleepiness in a snorer are often due to OSA. The oximetry sleep study in a symptomatic OSA patient often shows a characteristic repetitive oxygen desaturation pattern. However, a normal oximetry sleep study in a patient with suspected OSA cannot rule out UARS. It requires demonstration of snoring/upper airway resistance-related arousals on a PSG or a pragmatic approach of a therapeutic trial of CPAP.

However, a negative screening sleep study in a sleepy snorer and failure of response to a therapeutic trial of CPAP should lead to consideration of another diagnosis. Abnormal/frequent movements during sleep due to neurological disorders, such as periodic limb movement disorders, can cause sleep disruption and arousals. It is not uncommon for OSA and PLMS to coexist. It has been suggested that treatment of OSA with CPAP may precipitate unmasking of underlying PLMS. These patients have persistent daytime sleepiness, despite treatment of OSA with CPAP. Therefore, PLMS should be considered as a possible cause of persistent daytime sleepiness in OSA.

2. What are the common movement disorders during sleep?

The movement disorders during sleep can be due to a trivial cause, such as muscle jerks (hypnic jerks at sleep onset) or paralysis on awakening (sleep paralysis). However, they can be manifestations of serious underlying neurological disorders, such as Parkinson's disease, dementia or PLMS. During REM sleep there is complete muscle atonia; however, abnormal muscle activity during sleep can cause sleep talking, teeth grinding (bruxism) or sleep walking (somnambulism) in patients with REM sleep disorders.

3. What is PLMS?

PLMS, also known as nocturnal myoclonus, is a relatively common movement disorder during sleep and affects 4% of adults. It has a much higher prevalence in the elderly, especially females (11%). It causes characteristic repetitive flexion/extension movement of limbs during sleep, mainly legs (kicking) every 30 seconds or so, lasting for about 2–3 seconds. Each movement results in the brain or body waking up, with resultant sleep disruption and fragmentation. Anterior tibialis muscle EMG recording on PSG provides confirmation of the diagnosis (Figure 22.3). A typical pattern of repetitive leg kicking movements can also be seen on video recording (particularly on fast forwarding) during sleep. The description of the state of the bed sheets by the patient or partner of the movements during sleep may also provide a clue to the diagnosis. However, most patients are unaware of kicking their legs during sleep, but wake up unrefreshed from their sleep and feel sleepy during the daytime. Some of these patients may have associated neurological disorders, such as Parkinson's disease or narcolepsy. Similarly, factors such as shift work, exercise prior to sleep, use of benzodiazepine hypnotics, coffee drinking and snoring can increase the risk of PLMS.

Learning points

PLMS can cause symptoms similar to OSA in a snorer, coexist with OSA or be unmasked by the treatment of OSA with CPAP.

Clues to diagnosis may be provided by the partner's report of being kicked during sleep or the state of the bed sheets in the morning.

The stereotypical repetitive periodic kicking movements are seen on sleep video recording and PSS demonstrating leg movements associated with arousals, which provide confirmation of the diagnosis.

PLMS is a common condition and responds well to clonazepam in most patients.

Further reading

Merlino G, Gigli GL. Sleep-related movement disorders. Neurol Sci 2012 Jun;33(3): 491–513.

Walters AS. Clinical identification of the simple sleep-related movement disorders. Chest 2007 Apr;131(4):1260–6. Review.

Case 23
Worrying pauses in breath without choking and snoring— Central Sleep Apnoea

A 70-year-old newspaper editor's wife was concerned about pauses in his breath for two months. She did not hear him snore or have any choking episodes. He reported no sleep disturbance, but it was not refreshing. He felt tired and sleepy during the daytime. He had coronary artery bypass graft surgery three years ago and refractory congestive cardiac failure due to ischaemic cardiomyopathy and mitral regurgitation requiring cardiac resynchronization therapy (CRT) (implantable cardioverter defibrillator (ICD) with pacing capabilities (CRT-D)) two years ago. He reported a history of paroxysmal nocturnal dyspnoea that had improved with treatment of his heart failure. He had clinical features of congestive cardiac failure. He was a normal body weight of 73 kg for his height of 171 cm and neck size of 15.

His sleep study showed frequent episodes of central OSA, with an AHI of 37.3 (Figure 23.1). Airflow pattern was of crescendo–decrescendo breathing followed by prolonged apnoea and absent thoracoabdominal movements during apnoea (Cheyne–Stokes/periodic breathing) (Figure 23.2). The longest apnoea was for 64 seconds without thoracoabdominal movements/respiratory effort (central apnoeas). The apnoeas were associated with frequent oxygen desaturation, the SaO_2 dip rate was high at 32.4/hour and mean SaO_2 of 92.4, and a TST <90% of 28%. AHI consisted of 76% central apnoeas, 3% of obstructive apnoea and 17% mixed apnoeas. He was fitted with a nasal CPAP mask and received a trial of auto-CPAP. His wife reported no change in his apnoeas during sleep, despite good compliance with CPAP, and the patient noticed

Sleep Summary

Apnea/Hypopnea
    Index Time: 436.4 minutes
    Apnea + Hypopnea (A+H):   271   37.3 / h
    Supine A+H: 47   40.3 / h
    Non-Supine A+H: 224   36.7 / h

Position
    Supine Time: 69.9 minutes   16.0 %
    Non-Supine Time: 366.5 minutes   84.0 %
    Upright Time: 2.1 minutes   0.5 %
    Movement Time: 14.2 minutes   3.3 %

Oxygen Saturation
    Average Oxygen Saturation: 92.4 %
    Oxygen Desaturation Events (OD): 236   32.4 / h

Snoring
    Snore Time: 2.2 minutes   0.5 %
    Number of Snoring Episodes: 13

Apnea/Hypopnea Statistics

Respiration	Number	%	A or H/h	Supine	Non-Supine	Mean [seconds]	Longest [seconds]
Apnea	259	95.6	35.6	44	215	33.6	63.8
Obstructive	8	3.0	1.1	2	6	14.7	29.8
Central	205	75.6	28.2	39	166	32.9	63.8
Mixed	46	17.0	6.3	3	43	39.8	52.5
Hypopnea	12	4.4	1.6	3	9	22.9	44.2
Total	271		37.3	47	224	33.1	63.8

Fig. 23.1 Sleep study summary showing AHI, oxygen saturations and snoring data.

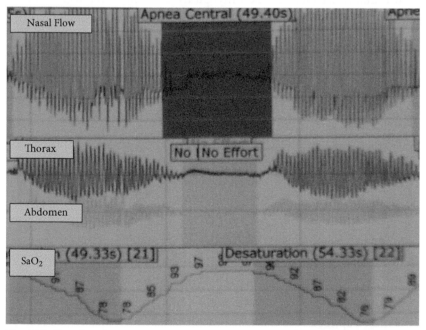

Fig. 23.2 Showing characteristic CSA pattern: absent nasal flow (apnoea) preceded and followed by crescendo–decrescendo flow pattern (Cheyne–Stoke breathing) with no effort on thoracic and abdominal effort and oxygen desaturation.

no change in his sleep quality and daytime symptoms. A sleep study on CPAP confirmed persistent CSA. Therefore, he was treated with servo-ventilation, which resulted in complete elimination of apnoeas during sleep with an improvement in sleep quality, daytime tiredness and sleepiness.

Questions

1 What is CSA?

2 How does heart failure cause CSA?

3 How do you treat CSA?

Answers

1. What is CSA?

CSA occurs when the brain fails to send an appropriate signal to the respiratory muscles to breathe. Patients with CSA make no effort to breathe during apnoea, as opposed to OSA when the brain sends much stronger signals to the respiratory muscle to breathe to overcome obstruction to the upper airway.

CSA is much less common than OSA, but can cause sleep disturbance and chronic intermittent hypoxia similar to OSA. Typical patients with CSA have witnessed apnoeas, but without any snoring or choking episodes. The recurrent apnoeas during sleep cause recurrent oxygen desaturation, and poor sleep quality and unrefreshing sleep. They also differ in physical characteristics from OSA patients and are of normal body weight and neck size, craniofacial appearance and oral cavity size. Furthermore, CSA is often seen in older men (>65 years) who have associated heart or cerebrovascular disease.

A characteristic type of breathing pattern—a gradual increase in breathing effort and rate followed by a decrease (crescendo–decrescendo) and complete cessation of breath (apnoea)—is known as Cheyne–Stokes respiration (CSR)/periodic breathing. The typical cycle of crescendo–decrescendo breathing followed by apnoea lasts for 30 seconds. Three such consecutive cycles with AHI of >5 for a 10-minute period of crescendo–decrescendo breathing is sufficient for the diagnosis of CSA. These patients have unstable respiratory drive. The common causes of this type of CSA include congestive cardiac failure, high altitude and cerebrovascular disorders.

CSA should be distinguished from 'pseudo CSA' in patients with respiratory muscle weakness/paralysis with OSA. They are unable to move their chest or abdomen (absent thoracoabdominal movement) during apnoeas and it is recorded as CSA. Monitoring of changes in intrathoracic pressure during respiration with an oesophageal balloon can help with accurate differentiation between CSA and OSA in patients with muscle weakness.

A few patients with OSA have a mixed pattern of CSA and OSA. Treatment with CPAP unmasks CSA and the sleep remains fragmented. This type of apnoea is known as 'complex sleep apnoea' and defined as more than five central sleep apnoeas per hour on CPAP. It is obvious that this group of patients will not respond to CPAP and may contribute to CPAP non-compliance.

2. How does heart failure cause CSA?

CSA of CSR is most commonly seen in patients with congestive heart failure—40–50% of heart failure patients may have such a breathing pattern. The CSA in patients with congestive heart failure is thought to be due to cerebral hypoxia and long circulatory time leading to elevated hypercapnic ventilatory response and an unstable ventilatory control system (enhanced loop gain). They tend to have faster breathing (hyperventilation) and hypocapnia during the daytime; however, hypocapnia as a result of hyperventilation during sleep reduces respiratory drive, leading to apnoeas. CSR due to CSA increases morbidity and mortality due to congestive cardiac failure. These patients often have advanced congestive cardiac failure and are on maximum medical treatment. Correction of CSR–CSA can not only improve their sleep quality, daytime fatigue and tiredness, but also their outcome. This is also seen in patients who have had a stroke or chronic renal failure.

3. How do you treat CSA?

Various different types of treatments have been attempted in patients with CSA from respiratory stimulants, such as theophylline, acetazolamide, oxygen and ventilatory devices.

In patients with primary CSA or CSA due to high altitude, respiratory stimulants such as acetazolamide and theophylline may be effective in improving sleep quality and apnoea. Often these measures fail, and treatment with oxygen and CPAP is required.

Theophylline increases adenosine levels and stimulates respiration. Although it has been shown to reduce CSA in small trials, it is not used often due to its narrow therapeutic margin and side effects.

Acetazolamide is a mild diuretic and, through its effect in inducing mild metabolic acidosis, stimulates respiration. It has been shown to improve CSA associated with high altitude.

In patients with CSA of the CSR type, optimization of heart failure treatment improves CSA. However, they are often on maximum medical treatment and on a waiting list for heart transplant. Overnight oxygen improves their sleep quality and periodic breathing in some of these patients—the exact mechanism of how oxygen works is not clear. CPAP if often effective and should be considered as an initial treatment option. CPAP improves sleep quality, nocturnal hypoxia, left ventricular function and exercise tolerance. Long-term CPAP can reduce the need for cardiac transplantation and the risk of mortality. However, in some patients, CSA, though improved, persists despite CPAP. These patients may benefit from BiPAP ventilation. A new type of ventilatory support device called adaptive servo-ventilation (ASV) measures the patient's flow (apnoea) and adjusts the delivery of pressure, abolishing apnoeas. This method of treatment has been shown to be more effective in suppressing CSA than CPAP. It should be considered in patients who show no or suboptimal response to CPAP.

Learning points

Suspect CSA as a cause of witnessed apnoeas in patients with no history of snoring or choking episodes during sleep.

Overnight oximetry sleep study cannot distinguish between CSA and OSA—simultaneous measurement of thoracoabdominal movement is required.

Advanced heart failure is one of the most common causes of CSA. These patients have characteristic waxing and waning breathing followed by apnoeas—known as periodic breathing/CSR.

Most patients with CSA of the CSR type can be treated with CPAP. However, a few require ASV.

Further reading

Malhotra A, Owens RL. What is central sleep apnea? Respir Care 2010;55(9):1168–78.

Case 24
Irresistible daytime sleepiness in a young obese woman

A 28-year-old office worker was referred by her GP because of long-standing snoring and a two-year history of waking up regularly at night and excessive sleepiness during the daytime at work. She could not control her sleepiness and slept at work for about 30 minutes every day. Previously, her job involved working irregular hours in a shift over a period of four years. Her father was diagnosed to have OSA and was on CPAP treatment at a sleep clinic. She had a tonsillectomy and adenoidectomy at 1 year of age.

She has had a long-standing battle with her obesity and managed to lose only 15 kg with stringent dieting and orlistat (xenical) tablets. She was on a waiting list for bariatric surgery. Her periods were irregular. She had poorly controlled asthma and continued to smoke one cigarette a day.

Review in the sleep clinic confirmed that she was excessively sleepy during the daytime, affecting her work; the ESS score was high at 16/24. Her sleep was disturbed; she went to bed at 10.30 in the evening and took a variable amount of time to fall asleep, and woke up three hours later followed by fragmented sleep until 7.00 in the morning. The description of her snoring was atypical, and it was more noisy and heavy breathing than snoring. There was no history of witnessed apnoea. She was obese with a BMI of 47, but maintained her neck size at 39 cm. An overnight oximetry sleep study was normal, with a normal mean SaO_2 of 95.5% and a dip rate of 0.4/hour.

Her clinical picture could not be explained on the basis of OSA.

Questions

1 What will you do next?

2 What is the probable diagnosis and how will you confirm the diagnosis?

3 What is the cause of narcolepsy?

4 How do you treat narcolepsy?

A family history of narcolepsy and the presence of a narcolepsy-associated gene, such as HLADR2, provides further support to the diagnosis. However, confirmation of the diagnosis requires a detailed PSG and measurement of daytime sleepiness with a multiple sleep latency test to demonstrate quick onset of sleep (reduced sleep latency) and entering into REM sleep straightaway (sleep onset REM).

Her EDS and cataplexy were suggestive of narcolepsy. She was prescribed modafinil (provigil) to help her daytime sleepiness. This helped her to stay awake at work until 3.00 in the afternoon, but she felt sleepy afterwards. Her blood test for the narcolepsy-associated HLA gene was negative. The neurologist agreed that her clinical picture was in keeping with a diagnosis of narcolepsy, though negative HLA was unusual, particularly in narcolepsy associated with cataplexy. In view of her marked obesity, EDS and irregular periods, an MRI head scan was performed to exclude primary hypothalamic disorder. A PSG and MSLT confirmed the diagnosis of narcolepsy. Her cataplexy was treated with clomipramine.

3. What is the cause of narcolepsy?

The cause of narcolepsy is not known, but brain (hypothalamus) neuropetide hypocretin levels are low.

The exact cause of narcolepsy is not known, but research over the last decade has shown that hypocretin (excitatory neuropeptide involved in the regulation of muscle tone) levels are low in the hypothalamus and cerebrospinal fluid (CSF). Hypocretin deficiency is thought to cause obesity as well. Rarely, narcolepsy associated with marked obesity and other endocrine dysfunction can be due to an anatomical lesion affecting the hypothalamus, such as craniopharyngioma. A normal MRI brain scan in our patient who had narcolepsy associated with obesity and irregular periods excluded such a lesion.

4. How do you treat narcolepsy?

Modafinil, a brain stimulant which improves daytime sleepiness, and clomipramine, a tricyclic antidepressant which controls cataplexy.

Modafinil is a short-acting CNS (central nervous system) stimulant with a low risk of dependence and improves daytime sleepiness for about four hours. Thus, taken twice a day at 8.00 a.m. and 12.00 noon can restore daytime alertness and function. It is safe except in patients with poorly controlled hypertension and reduced effectiveness of the oral contraceptive pill. Clomipramine, a tricyclic antidepressant, is the mainstay in the treatment of cataplexy and mainly works by suppressing REM sleep.

Learning points

For clinical features of OSA, but no evidence in the sleep study: reassess clinical features for an alternative diagnosis!

Uncontrollable daytime sleepiness affecting work in a young woman with no OSA: is it due to narcolepsy?

The cause of narcolepsy is not known, but brain (hypothalamus) neuropeptide hypocretin levels are low.

Modafinil, a brain stimulant which improves daytime sleepiness, and clomipramine, a tricyclic antidepressant which controls cataplexy.

Further reading

Ahmed I, Thorpy M. Clinical features, diagnosis and treatment of narcolepsy. Clin Chest Med 2010 Jun;31(2):371–81. Review.

Snoring and OSA: Role of dental and ENT surgeons

Case 25
Contribution of facial skeletal pattern to sleep apnoea

A 44-year-old male reported EDS and unrefreshing sleep. He was a shift worker, but felt that his sleep was poor and he woke up feeling unrefreshed and tired, which in turn made daytime functioning very difficult. His wife was unable to tolerate the snoring and they slept separately.

The patient was originally referred by his GP for a sleep assessment to a respiratory sleep service and diagnosed to have severe OSA on overnight PSG—his AHI was recorded as 65.5/per hour. An evaluation of his daytime sleepiness using ESS revealed excessive hypersomnia, with a score of 23 (maximum score 24). The patient's BMI revealed that he was obese (BMI = 33 kg/m^2). As a result, the patient was initially treated with an intelligent form of CPAP, but found tolerance to be difficult and that his symptoms persisted. As a result, he was seen by an ENT surgeon for further evaluation. The patient underwent a sleep nasendoscopy examination, which revealed predominately base of tongue obstruction to be taking place during the induced-phase of sleep (Pringle and Croft, 1993). This was also observed to improve when the mandible was postured forward (Johal et al., 2005).

The patient was subsequently referred to an orthodontist for specialist care in relation to the provision of an MAS.

Clinical examination revealed the patient was partially dentate in both jaws, with a number of teeth missing from his posterior dentition. There were a number of bridges present to replace the absent teeth. The periodontal health of the dentition was good, with no signs of active inflammation. Assessment of the temporomandibular joints (TMJ) revealed a good range of movement, with bilateral clicking of the joints on wide opening. Importantly, there were no symptoms of TMJ dysfunction.

Radiographic examination confirmed the clinical absence of teeth and large restorations, with extensive root treatments, and the presence of good levels of bone support in relation to the remaining dentition. Cephalometric skeletal evaluation revealed a degree of bimaxillary retrusion being present. This was most notable in relation to the posterior positioning of the mandible. Soft tissue, pharyngeal evaluation revealed a very narrow pharyngeal airway (Figure 25.1).

In view of the sleep nasendoscopy and cephalometric findings, both confirming the retro-positioning of the mandible, with subsequent tongue-base obstruction and narrowed pharyngeal airway, the patient was provided with a custom-made MAS. The MAS of choice was a removable Herbst appliance, which permitted incremental advancement of the mandible to be performed, in conjunction with technical support and limited mouth opening during sleep, with the use of inter-maxillary elastics (Figure 25.2).

The patient was subsequently reviewed and the splint adjusted in order to achieve maximum therapeutic effect, with further advancement provided. The MAS was well tolerated, and the patient initially attempted

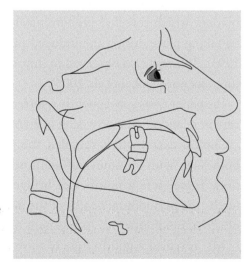

Fig. 25.1 Cephalometric tracing demonstrating the underlying skeletal anatomy contributing to the narrowed pharyngeal airway. Both the maxilla and mandible are retro-positioned before surgery.

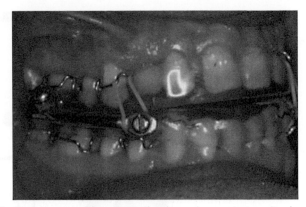

Fig. 25.2 The Herbst removable MAS, with telescopic arms to permit advancement of the mandible and the use of inter-maxillary elastics to limit mouth opening during sleep (from Johal and Battagel, 1999).
Source: Reprinted by permission from Maney, from 'An Investigation into the Changes in Airway Dimension and the Efficacy of Mandibular Advancement Appliances in Subjects with Obstructive Sleep Apnoea' in Journal of Orthodontics, Amandeep Johal and Joanna M. Battagel, 26: 205–210 (c) 1999.

to utilize it in conjunction with the CPAP. However, this proved difficult and the MAS was used in isolation, with reported improvement in symptoms, but not complete resolution. The patient returned 9 months later having lost some further posterior teeth through apical infection and reporting the fit of the MAS as being poor. The patient expressed he was very keen to explore the option of a surgical jaw correction as a long-term solution.

In view of the confirmed skeletal pattern, demonstrating that both the maxilla and, to a greater extent, the mandible were retro-positioned relative to the cranial base, the patient was planned for bimaxillary facial surgery to advance the maxilla by 5 mm and the mandible by 8 mm (Figure 25.3a and b). The patient reported significant improvement in his symptoms and a follow-up sleep study revealed a reduction in the AHI to ten episodes/hour.

Unfortunately, the patient found his symptoms returned and sought to have a new dental sleep appliance. In light of this, a custom-made medical dental sleep appliance was fabricated, which permitted self-adjustment of the degree of mandibular protrusion and complete limited mouth

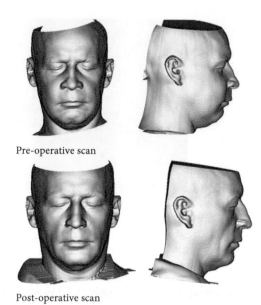

Pre-operative scan

Fig. 25.3a The cephalometric change observed in the maxilla and mandible following bimaxillary surgery.

Post-operative scan

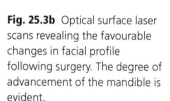

Fig. 25.3b Optical surface laser scans revealing the favourable changes in facial profile following surgery. The degree of advancement of the mandible is evident.

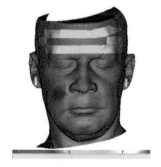

opening during sleep (medical dental sleep appliance (MDSA)) (Barnes et al., 2004; Figure 25.4). The patient reports following adjustment for maximum advancement, that he satisfactorily wears the MAS seven nights per week and between six and eight hours per night, with complete resolution of his symptoms. He remains on long-term review.

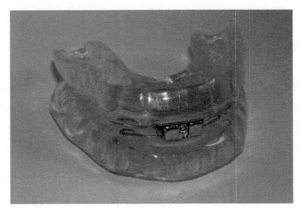

Fig. 25.4 The Mmcal dental sleep appliance permits self-adjustment of the degree of mandibular advancement and complete limited mouth opening during sleep.

Questions

1 What is the value of sleep nasendoscopy in MAS selection?

2 What type of follow-up measures would be appropriate for a patient with severe sleep apnoea being treated with MAS therapy?

3 How can the facial skeletal pattern of OSA patients be assessed? List two such findings.

Answers

1. What is the value of sleep nasendoscopy in MAS selection?

The sleep nasendoscopy permits a dynamic evaluation of the pharyngeal airway, in a state that 'mimics' sleep and permits an assessment of the site of collapse and the effect on both the airway collapse and snoring whilst performing simulated mandibular advancement.

2. What type of follow-up measures would be appropriate for a patient with severe sleep apnoea being treated with MAS therapy?

Subjective measures: daytime sleepiness (ESS); impact on snoring and compliance measure.

Objective measures: follow-up sleep study with the MAS in situ.

3. How can the facial skeletal pattern of OSA patients be assessed? List two such findings.

A cephalogram is indicated and subsequent analysis may reveal: maxillary retrusion; mandibular retrusion; reduced intermaxillary space; reduced anterior cranial base length.

Learning points

CPAP remains the gold standard treatment of choice in patients with severe obstructive sleep apnoea hypopnoea syndrome (OSAHS). Unfortunately, tolerance can be low. MAS therapy has now an increasingly recognized role and is the alternative method of choice in those patients who fail to tolerate CPAP therapy.

It is important that patients with OSAHS are appropriately followed up to ensure therapeutic success in the form of an overnight sleep study and subjective questionnaires.

Patients wishing to be considered for maxilla-facial surgery to address their OSASH should demonstrate an underlying skeletal discrepancy, and in particular mandibular retro-positioning. The use of an MAS to show improvement in symptoms permits a better prediction of surgical outcome. Long-term benefits of surgery may not be sustained.

MAS therapy can be considered in conjunction with CPAP therapy to ensure greater therapeutic effect and may permit lower CPAP pressures to be used.

Further reading

Barnes M, McEvoy RD, Banks S, Tarquinio N, Murray CG, Vowles N, Pierce RJ. Efficacy of positive airway pressure and oral appliance in mild to moderate obstructive sleep apnea. Am J Respir Crit Care Med 2004;170(6):656–64.

Johal, A, Arya D, Winchester LJ et al. The effect of a mandibular advancement splint in subjects with sleep-related breathing disorders. Br Dent J 2005;199(9):591–6.

Johal, A, Battagel JM. An investigation into the changes in airway dimension and the efficacy of mandibular advancement appliances in subjects with Obstructive Sleep Apnoea. Br J Orthod 1999;26:205–10.

Pringle MB, Croft CB. A grading system for patients with obstructive sleep apnoea based on sleep nasendoscopy. Clin Otolaryngol 1993;18:480–4.

Case 26
MAS therapy for severe OSAHS

A 31-year-old, otherwise fit and healthy male presented having being diagnosed with severe OSA. His principle complaints were loud disruptive snoring, which was adversely affecting his marriage, and the constant feeling of being tired and drained of energy to the extent that he was no longer able to concentrate at work. The patient compared the feeling to waking up in the morning having drunk two bottles of red wine the night before. He had seen his GP, who had prescribed him antidepressants and referred him for a sleep assessment. The overnight sleep study revealed severe OSA, and the AHI was recorded as 64.5/per hour. An evaluation of his daytime sleepiness using ESS revealed excessive hypersomnia, with a score of 16 (maximum score 24). The patient's BMI was within normal limits (BMI = 25.3 kg/m^2). An initial ENT consultation resulted in the patient undergoing a nasal septoplasty and being prescribed a steroid nasal spray, from which he obtained little benefit. He was subsequently prescribed n-CPAP, which he used intermittently for three years, with reported difficulties tolerating the mask and only limited symptomatic relief.

The patient felt he could no longer continue with the CPAP therapy and found his way to me at the Department of Orthodontics, Institute of Dentistry, Queen Mary College, London by means of an Internet search for specialist care in relation to the provision of an MAS.

Clinical examination revealed the patient was fully dentate in both jaws, with only first premolars missing in all quadrants, following orthodontic treatment. The patient had a Class III incisor relationship with a reduced overjet (2 mm) and overbite (1.5 mm). Periodontal health of the dentition was very good, with no signs of any active inflammation.

Assessment of the TMJ revealed a good range of movement, with no signs or symptoms of TMJ dysfunction.

A partner-recorded snoring questionnaire revealed significant disturbance, with the patient's wife reporting a poor quality of sleep for both herself and the patient, with very loud and frequent snoring and arrested breathing being experienced. Consequently, they were sleeping apart. An SF-36 quality of life questionnaire also revealed significant impacts in relation to both the energy/vitality and physical role limitation domains (Johal, 2006).

In order to ascertain a greater understanding of the aetiological basis of the airway collapse, a sleep nasendoscopy was performed. This revealed predominately base of tongue obstruction (Grade 5) to be taking place during the induced phase of sleep (Pringle and Croft, 1993). There was an observed improvement in both the snoring and airway patency when the mandible was postured forward (Johal et al., 2005).

In view of the sleep nasendoscopy findings, the patient was provided with a custom-made MAS. This was in the form of a medical dental sleep appliance and was fabricated, which permitted self-adjustment of the degree of mandibular protrusion and complete limited mouth opening during sleep (MDSA) (Barnes et al., 2004; Figure 26.1).

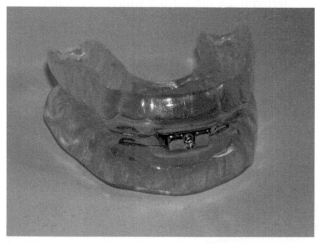

Fig. 26.1 The MDSA permits self-adjustment of the degree of mandibular advancement and complete limited mouth opening during sleep.

Following adjustment for maximum advancement, the patient reported that he satisfactorily wore the MAS seven nights per week for between six and eight hours per night. The patient reported how the appliance had 'transformed his life' and went on to say 'he had finally experienced his first night of proper sleep, waking in the morning feeling he had been born again'. Follow-up questionnaires demonstrated a very impressive improvement in his symptoms, including his partner's evaluation of his snoring, which she reported had completely resolved, and perhaps more importantly they were sharing the same bedroom. The ESS score was seen to reduce from 16 to 6. A follow-up overnight sleep study, undertaken with the MAS in place, revealed a significant improvement in the AHI score, reducing from 64.5 to 12.0 per hour. In addition, there was a significant reported improvement in relation to both the energy/vitality and physical role limitation domains.

He remains on long-term review.

Questions

1 What severity of OSA is recommended for the treatment with MAS therapy as a first-line choice?
2 Name two reported benefits of using the MDSA.

Answers

1. What severity of OSA is recommended for the treatment with MAS therapy as a first-line choice?

Patients with mild OSA, and moderate OSA patients if a preference for an MAS is expressed.

2. Name two reported benefits of using the MDSA.

It permits self-adjustment of the degree of mandibular advancement and complete limited mouth opening during sleep.

Learning points

The value of a customized MAS in terms of sustained use and patient comfort has been demonstrated over and above that achieved with cheaper 'boil and bite' prefabricated versions available via the Internet.

It is important that patients with moderate to severe OSAHS are appropriately followed up to ensure therapeutic success in the form of an overnight sleep study and subjective questionnaires.

Further reading

Barnes M, McEvoy RD, Douglas R, et al. Efficacy of positive airway pressure and oral appliance in mild to moderate obstructive sleep apnea. Am J Respir Crit Care Med 2004;170:656–64.

Johal A. Health-related quality of life in patients with sleep disordered breathing: effect of mandibular advancement appliances. J Prosthetic Dentistry 2006;96:298–302.

Johal A, Arya D, Winchester LJ et al. The effect of a mandibular advancement splint in subjects with sleep-related breathing disorders. Br Dent J 2005;199(9):591–6.

Pringle MB, Croft CB. A grading system for patients with obstructive sleep apnoea based on sleep nasendoscopy. Clin Otolaryngol 1993;18:480–4.

Case 27
Effectiveness, compliance and side effects of MAS therapy

A 33-year-old, otherwise fit and healthy male presented having being diagnosed with moderately severe OSA. His principle complaints were loud, disruptive snoring, which resulted in him and his wife sleeping in separate bedrooms and was adversely affecting his marriage, and daytime tiredness. He had seen his GP, who referred him for a sleep assessment at the ENT hospital. The overnight sleep study revealed moderate OSA, and an AHI was recorded as 20 per hour. An evaluation of his daytime sleepiness using ESS revealed excessive hypersomnia, with a score of 17 (maximum score 24). The patient's BMI was within normal limits (BMI = 25.9 kg/m^2). Sleep nasendoscopy revealed a sustained multi-segmental collapse of the pharyngeal airway (Grade 4) to be taking place during the induced phase of sleep (Pringle and Croft, 1993). There was an observed improvement in both the snoring and airway patency when the mandible was postured forward (Johal et al., 2005). Examination also revealed significant septal deviation and the patient underwent a septoplasty.

The patient was subsequently referred to the Department of Orthodontics, Institute of Dentistry, Queen Mary College, London for specialist care in relation to the provision of an MAS.

Clinical examination revealed the patient was fully dentate in both jaws, with the exception of the following teeth: first premolars and third molars in the maxilla, and second premolars in the mandible as a result of orthodontic treatment. The patient had a Class II division 1 incisor relationship with an increased overjet (5 mm) and overbite (4 mm). Periodontal health of the dentition was very good, with no signs of any active inflammation. Assessment of the TMJ revealed a good range of movement, with no signs or symptoms of TMJ dysfunction.

A partner-recorded snoring questionnaire revealed significant disturbance, with the patient's wife reporting a poor quality of sleep for both herself and the patient, with very loud and frequent snoring. Consequently,
they were sleeping apart. An SF-36 quality of life questionnaire also revealed
significant impacts in relation to the energy/vitality domain (Johal, 2006).

Treatment: In view of the sleep nasendoscopy findings, the patient was
provided with a custom-made mandibular advancement splint (MAS).
This was in the form of a medical dental sleep appliance and was fabricated, which permitted self-adjustment of the degree of mandibular
protrusion and complete limited mouth opening during sleep (MDSA)
(Barnes et al., 2004). Following adjustment for maximum advancement,
the patient reported that he satisfactorily wore the MAS seven nights per
week and for approximately six hours per night. The patient reported
significant improvement in his symptoms. Follow-up questionnaires
demonstrated a very impressive improvement in his symptoms. In the
partner's evaluation of his snoring, she reported a marked improvement, with mild to moderate snoring occurring on an occasional basis.
The ESS score was seen to reduce from 17 to 10. A follow-up overnight
sleep study, undertaken with the MAS in place, revealed a significant
improvement in the AHI score, reducing from 20 to 9.0 per hour. In
addition, there was a reported improvement in relation to the energy/
vitality domain of the SF-36 quality of life questionnaire.

The residual snoring is likely to be arising from soft palate involve-
ment, but the patient is not keen to undergo any pharyngeal surgery,
as he and his partner are happy with the present outcome. An objective evaluation of the patient's long-term (11 years) compliance with
MAS therapy was undertaken, using a microsensor thermometer (Figure 27.1) and revealed a high degree of use (seven days per week and an
average of seven hours per night).

A known long-term side effect of continued use of MAS therapy is
changes observed in the occlusion. These effects are evident in the patient's occlusion, with a reduction in the overjet (2 mm) and overbite
(1 mm) observed (Figure 27.2).

He remains on long-term review.

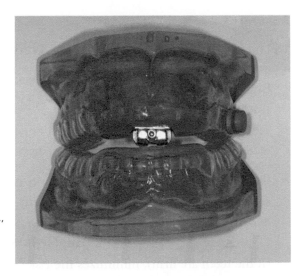

Fig. 27.1 Theramon objective adherence monitor attached to the MDSA.
Source: Reproduced from 'Objective measurement of sleep disordered breathing', Vanderverken O., Dieltjens, M., Wouters, K. et al, copyright © 2012 with permission from BMJ Publishing Group Ltd.

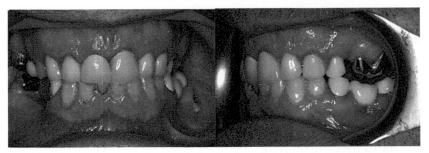

Fig. 27.2 Observed occlusal changes following long-term use of MAS therapy. (a) Frontal occlusal view; (b) Lateral occlusal view.

Questions

1 List one advantage and one disadvantage to a patient receiving a customised MAS, when compared to a 'boil and bite' prefabricated MAS.

2 What is the importance of ensuring patients have optimal dental health and asymptomatic TMJs prior to MAS therapy?

3 What dental measurements permit the dentist to monitor the development of any occlusal side effects?

Answers

1. List one advantage and one disadvantage to a patient receiving a customized MAS, when compared to a 'boil and bite' pre-fabricated MAS.

Advantage: improved fit and comfort (and compliance).

Disadvantage: requires a dentist to undertake mouldings of the teeth and consequently is more expensive.

2. What is the importance of ensuring patients have optimal dental health and asymptomatic TMJs prior to MAS therapy?

Optimal dental health ensures that the MAS will be better retained (if the teeth are firm), minimizes the risk of tooth movement from continued use and minimizes risk of tooth loss (if the periodontal health is less than optimal).

Symptomatic TMJs will only become more exacerbated and painful if the mandible is advanced to address the sleep-related breathing disorder.

3. What dental measurements permit the dentist to monitor the development of any occlusal side effects?

The overjet and overbite.

Learning points

It is important that informed consent is obtained and that the patient is made aware of the possibility of occlusal changes taking place following sustained use of their MAS.

Ensure the patient has optimal dental and periodontal health in the absence of any TJD prior to constructing an MAS.

Further reading

Barnes M, R McEvoy RD, Banks S, Tarquinio N, Murray CG, Vowles N, Pierce RJ. Efficacy of positive airway pressure and oral appliance in mild to moderate obstructive sleep apnea. Am J Respir Crit Care Med 2004; 170(6):656–64.

Johal, A. Health-related quality of life in patients with sleep disordered breathing: Effect of mandibular advancement appliances. J Prosthetic Dentistry 2006;96:298–302.

Johal A, Battagel JM, Kotecha BT. Sleep nasendoscopy: a diagnostic tool for predicting treatment success with mandibular advancement splints in obstructive sleep apnoea. Eur J Orthod 2005;27(6):606–614.

Pringle MB, Croft CB. A grading system for patients with obstructive sleep apnoea based on sleep nasendoscopy. Clin Otolaryngol 1993;18:480–4.

Vanderverken O, Dieltjens M, Wouters K, De Baker W, Van de Heyning P. Braem M. Objective measurement of sleep disordered breathing. Thorax 2013;68:91–6.

Case 28
Allergic rhinitis

A 45-year-old man was treated for severe OSA (AHI of 65) with overnight auto-pressure-adjusted CPAP for six months. He underwent a difficult course of treatment, and never tolerated the CPAP well. He had a BMI of 30. His ESS score was 15, which was improved marginally, having had a score of 17 before the start of CPAP treatment. He was using a full face mask, having had a history of significant bilateral nasal obstruction noted at the time of fitting a nasal CPAP mask. He reported long-standing nasal obstruction, and had previously undergone surgery on his nose, although he was not certain of the nature of that surgery. He had a past medical history of eczema, but was otherwise well. He worked as a shopkeeper. He was a non-smoker. There was no family history of nasal problems of which he was aware.

Questions

1 What nasal symptoms should be sought out when taking a history from this patient?
2 What investigations could you consider?
3 What steps would you recommend for allergen avoidance?
4 What pharmacological alternatives are there?
5 Why might the ESS be reduced?

Answers

1. What nasal symptoms should be sought out when taking a history from this patient?

Nasal symptoms to ask about include nasal obstruction, dripping from the nose (rhinorrhoea), decreased sense of smell (hyposmia), post-nasal drip, facial pressure and pain, sneezing, nasal itching, and itching or watering of the eyes. The time of day and the time of year of these symptoms is important, as are any notable exacerbating or alleviating factors, and whether the symptoms are unilateral or bilateral.

The patient reported perennial nasal obstruction and rhinorrhoea, particularly overnight and in the mornings. He reported sneezing and nasal itching, particularly at home and less so at work. There was no facial discomfort or eye symptoms, and the symptoms were symmetrical. The symptoms were notably better when he went on a beach holiday to Greece two years previously.

On examination, the nasal septum was in the midline, but the nasal mucosa was very pale and oedematous. There was a very limited nasal airway, and a significant amount of rhinorrhoea within the nasal cavity. Flexible nasendoscopic examination of the nose did not reveal polyps or any masses in the post-nasal space, but the view was limited by the extent of the nasal inflammation, and the rhinorrhoea within the nasal cavity (Figure 28.1). The pharynx was normal. He had a BMI of 30, with his weight distributed in an unremarkable fashion, and his collar size was 15.5 inches.

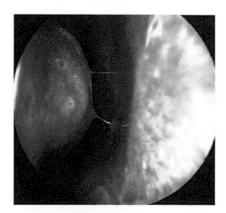

Fig. 28.1 Flexible nasendoscopy showing nasal inflammation and narrowing.

2. What investigations could you consider?

The history is highly suggestive of allergic rhinitis, although CPAP treatment itself can cause rhinitic changes and should be considered. The factors that are suggestive of allergy are the overtly allergic symptoms of itching, sneezing and eye watering, the history of eczema and the classically pale oedematous rhinitic changes within the nose.

Investigations should therefore be performed to investigate allergy. The most straightforward test is skin prick testing to known common aero-allergens. Skin prick testing involves introducing a small aliquot of a known allergen into the dermis using a small pin. A positive control using histamine and a negative control without any allergen is also required to validate the test. If the patient has been using antihistamines, this can mask positive results, but should also mask the positive histamine control. If the patient has an allergy to the testing materials, then the negative control should demonstrate an allergic response, which would also invalidate the test. Skin prick testing is relatively sensitive and specific, however it is fallible and, under certain circumstances, patients with negative skin prick testing may be treated as having allergic rhinitis (Figure 28.2).

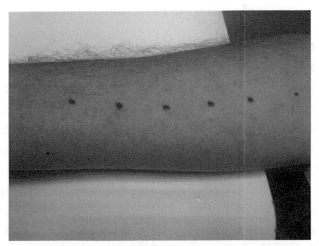

Fig. 28.2 Skin prick testing demonstrates allergy to house dust mites and cat hair.

Common aero-allergens include grass pollens, tree pollens, fungi, house dust mites, and pet hair, such as from cats and dogs. Less common allergens that may be seen in urban populations include cockroach droppings. His perennial history of allergic symptoms deteriorating overnight at home is most suggestive of a house dust mite allergy. There are recognized patterns of seasonal allergy that will vary dependent on the country, and to some extent the region in which you practise.

Alternatives to skin prick testing include blood tests for allergen-specific IgE, such as the radioallergosorbent test (RAST testing) which can identify allergens when skin prick testing may not be possible, for example, due to concerns over anaphylaxis, lack of specific allergens or if the patient has taken an antihistamine. RAST testing is less accurate than skin prick testing, with false positive results being relatively more common. Furthermore, the correlation between the extent of a response and clinical symptoms is less strong with RAST tests than with skin prick tests.

Further tests could include an objective measure of nasal patency, such as nasal inspiratory peak flows, rhinomanometry or acoustic rhinometry. Equally, in patients with less overtly allergic symptoms, CT imaging of the sinuses could be considered. Systemic allergic responses can be assessed with serum IgE levels and vitamin D can also be considered, as deficiency may exacerbate rhinitis.

3. What steps would you recommend for allergen avoidance?

Allergen avoidance is the first and most important step in the treatment of allergic rhinitis. Avoidance should concentrate on each of the identified stimuli. First, exposure to cat hair should be reduced. If the patient has a cat, then it may be possible for the pet to be rehomed. If this is not possible, then regular cleaning, and limits to areas in which the pet is kept, may be beneficial. Specifically, excluding the pet from the bedroom and indoor carpeted living areas is recommended.

House dust mite allergen exposure may be reduced by a number of factors in the bedroom and throughout the house. In the bedroom, cushions and mattresses can be covered with allergen-proof covers. Bedding and soft toys should be regularly washed at high temperatures (>60°C). Books, soft toys and thick curtains can also store dust mites and can be removed, with curtains being replaced by blinds. Throughout the house, but particularly in the bedroom, carpets can be replaced by hard floors. Any carpets in the household, and also furniture, should be hoovered regularly. Lastly, lowering indoor humidity—using air conditioning in the summer, and central heating in winter—can also help symptoms.

Grass and tree pollen allergens may be avoided by limiting time spent in grassy or wooded areas during the seasons in which that allergy is most prevalent. Fungal allergies may be managed similarly to the house dust mite allergy. Identifying triggers to the allergic symptoms may help identify avoidance tactics.

The patient already had hard floors, did not have a cat and regularly washed his sheets. He felt he had limited his exposure as much as he could. He asked about medications that may help him.

4. What pharmacological alternatives are there?

Different nasal medications may be effective in controlling different nasal allergic symptoms.

It is important to note that both the underlying sleep disordered breathing and the difficulty tolerating nasal CPAP may be manifestations of the nasal obstruction. Nasal obstruction is most effectively treated with topical nasal steroid. This may be in the form of sprays, such as fluticasone or mometasone, or in the form of drops. Drops may provide a much higher dose of topical steroid; however, some medications, such as betamethasone, may have significant systemic absorption, and protracted courses should be avoided. Topical steroids may also be effective for rhinorrhoea.

Systemic steroid is highly effective at treating these symptoms, but is contraindicated by its side effects. Nevertheless, patients with rheumatological disease may use steroids for other indications.

More allergic symptoms can be controlled with systemic antihistamines, such as cetirizine or loratadine. A topical antihistamine, azelastine, is effective for breakthrough symptoms. Rhinorrhoea can be treated with topical ipratropium bromide.

Fluticasone nasal drops and oral cetirizine controlled the patient's nasal and allergic symptoms very effectively. A further sleep study demonstrated that his severe OSA had significantly improved, with an AHI of 18. He continued to use his CPAP, and was able to change his full face mask for a nasal mask. His compliance improved significantly. He felt significantly less somnolent with an ESS score of 3.

5. Why might the ESS be reduced?

There are three reasons that the ESS may be reduced. The most obvious is the improved CPAP compliance. This may be due to the ability to use a nasal mask, or the improved nasal patency independent of the mask. Second, the AHI falling to a third of the previous level will mean that sleep quality is improved, even during periods when the CPAP is not used. Lastly, allergic rhinitis causes fatigue, and successfully treating the allergy may lead to a significant decrease in daytime somnolence independent of sleep quality. It is important to note possible confounding factors when assessing a patient's somnolence. Other conditions that may lead to fatigue and daytime somnolence include anaemia, rheumatological disease, chronic infections and some malignancies.

Learning points

The nasal airway is vital for efficient ventilation during sleep, and should be assessed in patients with sleep-disordered breathing.

Diagnoses of allergic rhinitis are principally clinical, with skin prick testing being a useful adjunct.

Management of allergic rhinitis depends initially on allergen avoidance, and subsequent pharmacotherapy.

Further reading

Brozek JL, Bousquet J, Baena-Cagnani CE et al. Allergic rhinitis and its impact on asthma (ARIA) guidelines: 2010 revision (Global Allergy and Asthma European Network) J Allergy Clin Immunol 2010 Sep;126(3):466–76.

Kotecha B. The nose, snoring and obstructive sleep apnoea. Rhinology 2011 Aug;49(3): 259–63.

Case 29
Nasal polyposis

A 43-year-old gentleman was referred to the ENT clinic by his GP, as his wife had been complaining of worsening snoring and had witnessed frequent apnoeas of 5–10 seconds. He had a past medical history of asthma. He had significant daytime somnolence. He complained of a number of unusual symptoms including nocturia, decreased libido and sleepwalking.

Questions

1 What may these unusual symptoms represent?

2 What would your next step be?

3 Prior to surgery, are there any investigations that would be recommended?

4 What does the CT scan show?

5 What are nasal polyps?

6 Why does nasal obstruction lead to sleep-disordered breathing in patients who mouth breathe comfortably when awake?

Answers

1. What may these unusual symptoms represent?

Given the context of witnessed apnoeas and snoring, sleep apnoea seemed likely. Sleep apnoea causes overnight hypoxia which leads to a systemic sympathetic response. This causes a number of symptoms including nocturia, enuresis, morning headache, decreased libido, nocturnal awakenings and sleepwalking.

He also complained of total loss of smell (anosmia) for the last six years, rhinorrhoea and near total nasal obstruction. On examination, there was a grade 3 nasal polyp on anterior rhinoscopy (Figure 29.1).

2. What would your next step be?

After completion of the history and examination, the question is whether to treat the nasal polyposis or investigate the sleep-disordered breathing in the first instance. This will depend on the chosen treatment for the nasal polyposis.

Should the polyps be unilateral, they should be investigated and biopsied in the operating theatre on an urgent basis.

Bilateral nasal polyposis can be treated with topical, or systemic, steroids, and surgery. One option would be to use a short course of

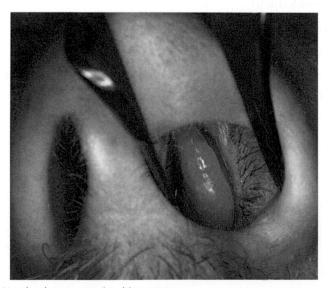

Fig. 29.1 Nasal polyp on anterior rhinoscopy.

oral steroid (five to seven days), and commence nasal steroid drops during this course. Smaller polyps may be treated with nasal drops alone or nasal sprays. However, in this case, where the polyps almost prolapse out of the nose, these are unlikely to be successful. Surgery in the form of endoscopic polypectomy is likely to be the best option.

If medical management is chosen, then the sleep disorder could be investigated. However, if surgical management is chosen, it may be prudent to defer a sleep study until surgery has been undertaken, as it is not likely to be representative of the quality of sleep once surgery has restored the nasal airway.

The patient was elected to undergo endoscopic polypectomy.

3. Prior to surgery, are there any investigations that would be recommended?

A CT scan of the sinuses would be recommended before endoscopic nasal surgery to guide surgery and define anatomical limits.

4. What does the CT scan show?

This is a coronal section of a CT through the anterior part of the ethmoid sinuses. All imaged sinuses are opacified, and there are bilateral polyps. On the right-hand side, the middle turbinate has a potential space within it (a concha bullosa) (Figure 29.2).

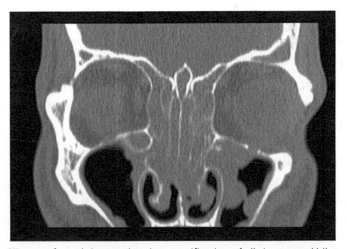

Fig. 29.2 CT scan of nasal sinuses showing opacification of all sinuses and bilateral nasal polyps.

The patient underwent endoscopic polypectomy, and his symptoms improved greatly. A sleep study demonstrated only mild OSA, with an AHI of 6.2.

5. What are nasal polyps?

Nasal polyps are polypoidal lumps of tissue comprised nasal mucosa. Their exact aetiology is unknown, although they are associated with a number of medical conditions, such as asthma, cystic fibrosis and Kartagener's syndrome.

6. Why does nasal obstruction lead to sleep-disordered breathing in patients who mouth breathe comfortably when awake?

During ventilation at rest, the nasal airway has less resistance than the oral airway. This is particularly marked during sleep, when relaxation of the pharyngeal and glossal musculature leads to a reduction in the retroglossal airway. This makes it relatively much less efficient to mouth breathe. Thus, nasal obstruction has a disproportionately large effect on the efficiency of ventilation during sleep.

Learning points

Nasal polyposis characteristically leads to hyposmia, rhinorrhoea and subsequently nasal obstruction. Facial pain or pressure are unusual symptoms in this population.

In bilateral nasal polyposis, CT scanning is only routinely used to guide a planned surgical procedure.

The mainstay of management of nasal polyposis is topical steroids. Short courses of systemic steroids and polypectomy are adjuncts to topical steroid treatment.

Further reading

Craig TJ, Ferguson BJ, Krouse JH. Sleep impairment in allergic rhinitis, rhinosinusitis, and nasal polyposis. Am J Otolaryngol 2008 May–Jun;29(3): 209–17.

Fokkens WJ, Lund VJ, Mullol J, et al. EPOS 2012: European position paper on rhinosinusitis and nasal polyps 2012. Rhinology 2012 Mar;50(1):1–12.

Case 30
Septoplasty

A 52-year-old man presented at clinic to talk about his CPAP. He had been treated for OSA with CPAP for 18 months. He initially used a nasal mask; however, the pressure was too high to be comfortable, and he changed to a full face mask. He found the face mask very uncomfortable to use, as it was pressing on his face around the mouth, and he was having leaks around this area.

Ever since an injury in his thirties, he had had nasal blockage, more on the left side than the right. He had no other nasal symptoms. He had grade 1 tonsils, and generally floppy pharyngeal mucosa. His Mallampati grade is 3, and he had a BMI of 36. His neck collar size was 18.5 inches.

Examination of the nose revealed a septum that was grossly deviated to the left side (Figure 30.1). The left inferior turbinate appeared oedematous and enlarged, but the nasal mucosa was otherwise normal.

Questions

1 Does the mucosa on the left inferior turbinate indicate underlying rhinitis?
2 What investigations could be considered?
3 Is his BMI a contraindication to surgery?
4 What are the complications of surgery?
5 Are there alternatives?
6 Is septoplasty likely to have any long-lasting effect on the underlying sleep-disordered breathing?

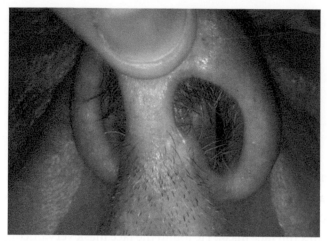

Fig. 30.1 Marked nasal septal deviation narrowing left nasal cavity.

Answers

1. Does the mucosa on the left inferior turbinate indicate underlying rhinitis?

It is possible that this mucosa indicates underlying rhinitis. The mucosa on the left is swollen, but is significant because it is reversible and may well return to normal when the airflow through the nose is re-established. The nasal obstruction may well be the cause rather than the result of rhinitis.

3. Is a BMI a contraindication to surgery?

The BMI of 36 was a relative contraindication to surgery. In this case, the benefits were sufficiently great for this to be overlooked. The

Answers

1. Does the mucosa on the left inferior turbinate indicate underlying rhinitis?

It is possible that this mucosa indicates underlying rhinitis. The inferior turbinate on the left may represent a significant proportion of the viewable nasal mucosa should visualization of the nose be limited by the septal deflection and the inferior turbinate. Nasal endoscopy could help to bypass this.

However, it is more likely that the inferior turbinate is enlarged as a result of the increased airflow on this side associated with the septal deflection. This is very commonly seen with significant septal deflections, and does not indicate an underlying rhinitic process.

2. What investigations could be considered?

It is important to quantify the extent to which he is using his CPAP. The length and frequency of CPAP use is recorded by many CPAP devices. Furthermore, the required CPAP pressures can be reviewed. Some CPAP devices will autoset the pressure, and these parameters can be downloaded from the device; this will give an objective measure of the difficulties with the CPAP treatment.

Nasal patency can be assessed using nasal inspiratory peak flow measurements; however, these are predominantly used to assess the result of treatment.

The relative patency of each side can be assessed using acoustic rhinometry; however, this is only rarely used in clinical practice, and usually an assessment based on clinical examination is sufficient. Mladina has proposed a grading system for septal deviation; however, once again, this is infrequently used in clinical practice.

Septoplasty surgery was recommended, and the patient indicated a willingness to undergo any procedure that may aid his use of CPAP.

3. Is his BMI a contraindication to surgery?

His BMI of 36 was a relative contraindication to surgery. In this case, the benefits were sufficiently great for this to be overlooked. The rationale for this being a contraindication was the relatively higher incidence of peri-operative and post-operative complications.

4. What are the complications of surgery?

Complications of septoplasty include infection, bleeding, septal perforation (which may lead to nasal crusting, epistaxis or even a 'saddle' deformity of the external nose), a loss of support of the nasal tip with a consequent impingement of the external nasal valve, failure to improve the nasal airway, numbness of the teeth and anosmia. General anaesthetic complications of surgery such as venous thromboembolism should also be considered.

5. Are there alternatives?

Alternatives to septoplasty include medical and other surgical treatments. Topical nasal steroid may lead to some improvement in nasal patency. This would be particularly relevant if there were significant rhinitic changes within the nose. However, CPAP rhinitis is something to consider, and given the small side effect profile of topical nasal steroids, they would be a reasonable conservative measure.

Surgical alternatives include reduction of the inferior turbinates, particularly on the unaffected side of the nose. This carries relatively less complications; however, it is much less likely to be successful in the long term, and may lead to scarring/adhesions/synechiae in the nose. If the external nasal pyramid is deviated, then to correct the septal deflection may require septorhinoplasty.

The patient underwent septoplasty, and was able to use his CPAP effectively and comfortably. His compliance increased notably, and his daytime somnolence decreased. He is maintained on CPAP treatment.

6. Is septoplasty likely to have any long-lasting effect on the underlying sleep-disordered breathing?

It is unlikely, but possible, that septoplasty in itself will 'cure' the OSA. A small proportion of patients with OSA can be definitively treated with nasal surgery. A larger proportion of patients with snoring can be definitively treated with nasal surgery, although this group still forms a minority of patients who snore. It is much more common for nasal complaints to be part of a clinical syndrome of OSA and, in these cases, treating the nasal complaint will not take the OSA away, but may potentiate the treatment of OSA with CPAP.

Learning points

Contralateral enlargement of the inferior turbinate is frequently seen in septal deviation.

Nasal obstruction can make it difficult to tolerate CPAP treatment.

In patients with nasal obstruction, it is important to consider rhinitis prior to surgery for structural nasal obstruction.

Further reading

Georgalas C. The role of the nose in snoring and obstructive sleep apnoea: an update. Eur Arch Otorhinolaryngol 2011 Sep;268(9):1365–73.

Poirier J, George C, Rotenberg B. The effect of nasal surgery on nasal continuous positive airway pressure compliance. Laryngoscope 2014 Jan;124(1):317–19.

Case 31
Upper airway resistance syndrome

A 56-year-old lady presented with snoring and daytime somnolence. Her ESS score was 14. She had no nasal obstruction, and her BMI was 29. Examination of the oropharynx revealed grade 2 tonsils. Examination was otherwise normal. She underwent overnight pulse oximetry which was reported as normal.

Questions

1 Does the overnight pulse oximetry exclude OSA?
2 What further information will this provide?
3 What is flow limitation, and what is its significance?
4 What investigations and treatments can be considered?

Answers

1. Does the overnight pulse oximetry exclude OSA?

Whilst overnight pulse oximetry is not the gold standard for the assessment of sleep apnoea, a normal study is highly unlikely in a patient with OSA. It should be ensured that an adequate recording was obtained and, if there is a significant clinical suspicion of OSA, then PSG or multichannel sleep study can be performed.

An multichannel sleep study was arranged to reassess the sleep quality.

2. What further information will this provide?

There is a variety of ways of assessing sleep quality. Multichannel sleep study such Embletta includes pulse oximetry, measurement of the heart rate, recording of the volume of snoring, nasal airflow, flow limitation, recording respiratory effort, and chest and abdominal movement. The gold standard is PSG (although this term is used rather variably when describing sleep assessment), which usually includes EEG recordings to assess sleep stages. PSG can be used to assess conditions such as narcolepsy or atypical epilepsy. Embletta will give a more reliable measurement of upper airway obstruction than pulse oximetry. Furthermore, measurements of flow limitation can be important in sleep-disordered breathing.

The sleep study showed an AHI of 1.2, and a flow limitation index of 37.4%.

3. What is flow limitation, and what is its significance?

Flow limitation describes ventilation in which there is a period when there is no increase in flow, despite an increase in respiratory effort. This leads to a plateau when recording flow against pressure. There are a number of ways in which this can be measured. They include using oesophageal manometers to detect intrathoracic pressure. The least invasive measure is recording ventilator flow during the respiratory cycle. 'Plateaus' in flow on inspiration are abnormal—usually, the ventilator flow pattern is sinusoidal. High numbers of breaths with evidence of flow limitation are highly suggestive of UARS.

This condition is characterized by respiratory effort related arousals (RERAs). In this syndrome, a patient does not succumb to apnoeas with their reversible upper airway obstruction, but rather arouses themselves with the effort of inspiration to overcome the obstruction. The presentation is thus similar to OSA.

The patient was diagnosed with UARS, and asked what her options for treatment were.

4. What investigations and treatments can be considered?

Similarly to the assessment of the upper airway for OSA, the assessment of the entire upper airway is indicated. This can be done through imaging, endoscopy, sleep nasendoscopy or an apnoeagraph. This allows treatment to be targeted to areas that are likely to be implicated in the UARS.

The patient was investigated using an apnoeagraph, which indicated obstruction around the level of the nasopharynx and oropharynx. The patient opted for surgical management, and underwent tonsillectomy and laser-assisted uvulopalatoplasty (LAUP). On follow-up three months later, her sleep quality had notably improved, and her ESS score had decreased to 5.

Learning points

PSG including video and EEG monitoring is the gold standard for assessment of sleep; however, it is expensive.

Sleep-disordered breathing can lead to the symptoms of OSA even in the absence of apnoeas and hypopnoeas.

UARS is managed in a similar fashion to mild OSA.

Further reading

Iber C, Ancoli-Israel S, Chesson AL, et al. The AASM manual for the scoring of sleep and associated events: rules, terminology and technical specifications. American Academy of Sleep Medicine 2007.

Pépin JL, Guillot M, Tamisier R, Lévy P. The upper airway resistance syndrome. Respiration 2012;83(6):559–66.

This condition is characterized by respiratory effort related arousals (RERAs). In this syndrome, a patient does not present with apnoeas with their reversible upper airway obstruction, but rather as-
sociates themselves with the effort of breathing it as to maintain their
attention. The presentation is similar to obstructive sleep apnoea.

The patient was diagnosed with UARS, and it was clear that the
obstructive process was present.

Case 32
Laser Assisted Uvulopalatoplasty (LAUP)/tonsillectomy

A 42-year-old man with OSA had been treated with a CPAP machine at 17 cm of water using a nasal mask for the last two years, but had poor compliance with treatment. He was unable to tolerate wearing the mask for any length of time, and found the high pressure gave him a suffocating feeling and forced air out of his mouth. He had a BMI of 33. He was known to be hypertensive, for which he took lisinopril.

Questions

1 Approximately what proportion of patients prescribed CPAP do not use the treatment?
2 What measures could you try with the patient to attempt to improve his compliance with CPAP?
3 What does his sleep study show?
4 What are the options for management?
5 Which investigations could help assess this patient to see if there is a relevant surgical approach?
6 What are the potential disadvantages of surgical management in cases similar to this?

Answers

1. Approximately what proportion of patients prescribed CPAP do not use the treatment?

The term 'CPAP compliance' generally refers to use of the CPAP mask on four or more nights per week for four or more hours each night. Approximately 60–70% of patients prescribed CPAP reach this level of CPAP use.

2. What measures could you try with the patient to attempt to improve his compliance with CPAP?

You could try to increase his motivation by advising him of the effect of untreated OSA on his health—notably the increased risk of cardiac disease and stroke (especially in the context of his hypertension). You could also advise him of the benefits to his quality of life—less daytime somnolence, less nocturia, improved libido, and better memory and concentration.

You could give him advice about the use and care of the mask, and advise him to try a full face mask.

You could try to change his CPAP pressures to see if the AHI could be decreased sufficiently with lower pressures. Furthermore, an auto-pressure set CPAP device could be used.

You could advise him to lose weight, as that may decrease his CPAP pressure requirement and possibly mean he would not need CPAP. Medications such as orlistat may help with this.

You could ask him about nasal rhinitic symptoms. CPAP rhinitis can be treated with intranasal steroid.

Despite best efforts, the patient was still unable to use his CPAP regularly. He had significant daytime somnolence, and asked about his options.

He was diagnosed with OSA two years ago, at which time this was his sleep study:

3. What does his sleep study show?

This demonstrates OSA with a notable supine (positional) component (Figure 32.1).

*Somno*logica

Summary Graph

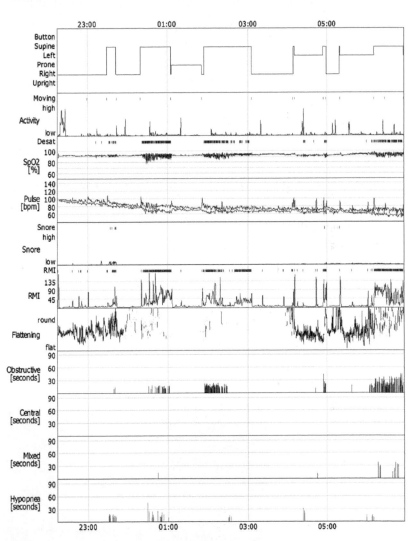

Fig. 32.1 Sleep study showing recurrent oxygen desaturation associated with obstructive apnoea notable in supine position.

4. What are the options for management?

There is a range of treatments that may be of benefit to him. First, there are devices used to prevent patients sleeping in a supine position. These are currently infrequently used, but have previously been popular. These may include balls strapped between the shoulder blades, alarms in the bed that detect when the patient lies on their back, or arranging the bed in such a way that turning is prevented.

Second, oral appliances such as mandibular advancement devices (MADs) may move the mandible and thus the tongue base anteriorly. This improves the pharyngeal airway and may treat the OSA.

Third, weight loss remains an option.

Fourth, there are surgical approaches to treat the obstruction. The supine element of OSA in this case may indicate that tonsillectomy would be advantageous.

On examination in clinic, the patient had minimal rhinitis associated with his CPAP use. There was no significant nasal obstruction, and this problem was well controlled with intranasal steroids. The septum was in the midline. There was no evidence of nasal polyposis. He had grade 3 tonsils (Figure 32.2), a floppy soft palate with redundant folds of mucosa, and a Mallampati score of 2. There was moderate adiposity in the neck. He was wearing an 18-inch collar.

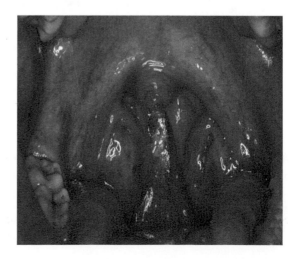

Fig. 32.2 Oral cavity showing enlarged tonsils (grade 3).

5. **Which investigations could help assess this patient to see if there is a relevant surgical approach?**

   Whilst clinically it sounds as though the patient's obstruction is most likely to be arising from his tonsils and soft palate, this can be investigated by a number of methods. These include sedation/sleep nasendoscopy, acoustic analysis of snoring, use of an 'apnoeagraph' pressure catheter and imaging of the upper respiratory tract.

   After undergoing sleep nasendoscopy, which confirmed inspiratory collapse in the palatal and oropharyngeal area, the patient underwent tonsillectomy and LAUP. A sleep study performed eight weeks post-operatively showed that the AHI had fallen from 20/hr to 5.6/hr.

6. **What are the potential disadvantages of surgical management in cases similar to this?**

   These operations carry significant risks; 5% of patients undergoing tonsillectomy have post-operative bleeding leading to readmission, and 1% undergo further surgery to stop this bleeding. These operations are very painful, and have a lower success rate than CPAP treatment in reducing episodes of apnoea. Other operative risks include the risk of infection, damage to the teeth, nasal regurgitation, a globus sensation and complications associated with anaesthesia.

   Whilst tonsils do not regrow, it is possible that over a long period of time the laxity of the soft palate may increase, and in a proportion of patients undergoing surgical management of their OSA, symptoms may recur.

Learning points

Tonsillar hypertrophy may cause significant airway obstruction during sleep-related pharyngeal relaxation.

Methods to assess the anatomy of obstruction in OSA include drug-induced sleep nasendoscopy, apnoeagraph devices and imaging of the upper airway.

Surgical management in the oropharynx is usually reserved for those patients who have been non-compliant with CPAP therapy.

Further reading

Borek RC, Thaler ER, Kim C et al. Quantitative airway analysis during drug-induced sleep endoscopy for evaluation of sleep apnea. Laryngoscope 2012 Nov;122(11): 2592–9.

Sawyer AM, Gooneratne NS, Marcus CL et al. A systematic review of CPAP adherence across age groups: clinical and empiric insights for developing CPAP adherence interventions. Sleep Med Rev 2011 Dec;15(6): 343–56.

Case 33
Epiglottic trapdoor

A 28-year-old man presented to his GP with daytime somnolence and witnessed sleep-disordered breathing. His partner reported episodes of apnoea followed by tachypnoea and apparent choking episodes. He had a BMI of 26, and was otherwise well. He had no nasal symptoms, and nasal and oropharyngeal examination was normal. He was referred to his local sleep unit, where PSG demonstrated severe OSA, with an AHI of 32. He was commenced on CPAP treatment and initially tolerated this well.

Five years later, during a routine CPAP appointment, he reported that he had been having more difficulties. His CPAP pressures had been high throughout his treatment, but after recent dental work he was having increasing leaks from the mouth, which woke him up. He was unable to tolerate a full face mask. He was using the CPAP increasingly less frequently. He asked whether there were any alternatives to CPAP treatment. Examination and daytime somnolence were unchanged.

Questions

1 What investigations would you consider?
2 What are the options for management?
3 Are there any potential side effects of this treatment that should be monitored?

Answers

1. What investigations would you consider?

It is possible that, over time, sleep parameters will change. Apnoea indexes are relatively likely to worsen over time (OSA is more common in an older age group). Furthermore, change of weight or redistribution of fatty tissue may change the sleep quality. A repeat sleep study could therefore be considered in order to quantify the extent of the sleep-disordered breathing at that time.

Anatomical assessment of the upper airway during sleep would allow the site (or sites) of obstruction to be ascertained. This could take the form of sleep nasendoscopy/drug-induced sleep endoscopy, imaging studies or an apnoeagraph.

Empirical management with an MAS is also an option to see if anterior movement of the mandible and the tongue base would improve the sleep-disordered breathing. Generally, these devices are able to move the tongue base 5–6 mm anteriorly.

An MAS was well tolerated, but produced no improvement in symptoms. The patient underwent sleep nasendoscopy. During the sleep nasendoscopy, it was clear that the point of obstruction was at the epiglottis. The epiglottis prolapsed with inspiration such that the tip pressed against the posterior pharyngeal wall, and the body of the epiglottis obstructed the retroglossal airway almost totally. This is referred to as 'epiglottic trapdoor phenomenon'.

2. What are the options for management?

CPAP treatment could be persevered with. An MAS had failed, but more definitive movement of the mandible and maxilla in the form of mandibular maxillary advancement could be considered. Wedge excision of the midline of the epiglottis was also an option.

The patient opted to undergo wedge excision of the epiglottis. The procedure was uneventful, and improved the sleep-disordered breathing significantly. A sleep study performed four months postoperatively demonstrated that the AHI had decreased to 2.3, and the patient was significantly less somnolent.

3. **Are there any potential side effects of this treatment that should be monitored?**

The epiglottis is most important for the prevention of aspiration during swallowing. Whilst this role is frequently overestimated (the tongue base is relatively much more important in preventing aspiration), the possibility of significant aspiration is something that should be closely monitored. Suspected aspiration can be assessed using a flouroscopic water-soluble contrast swallow.

Learning points

OSA may occur as a result of obstruction at any point in the upper airway.

Obstruction at the tongue base can be managed with CPAP, a MAD/MAS or surgically.

A balance has to be made between maintaining the airway during sleep and preserving pharyngeal structures that are important in swallowing.

Further reading

Li KK. Hypopharyngeal airway surgery. Otolaryngol Clin North Am 2007 Aug;40(4): 845–53.

Marklund M, Verbraecken J, Randerath W. Non-CPAP therapies in obstructive sleep apnoea: mandibular advancement device therapy. Eur Respir J 2012 May;39(5): 1241–7.

Case 34
Tracheostomy

A 52-year-old female patient presented to her GP with a 'globus' or foreign body feeling in the throat accompanied by snoring and witnessed disordered breathing overnight.

Questions

1 Which of these symptoms is more concerning?
2 What is the next stage for her management?
3 What are the options for management of the sleep disorder?
4 What tracheostomy care advice should she be given?
5 What are the potential complications of tracheostomy?

Answers

1. Which of these symptoms is more concerning?

Globus sensation is a common symptom characterized by a feeling of there being a foreign body within the throat. It is not associated with head and neck cancer, and is not thought as a 'red flag' symptom which would warrant urgent referral to head and neck cancer services. Causes include conditions such as gastro-oesophageal reflux disease (GORD) (or laryngo-pharyngo reflux (LPR)). Sleep-disordered breathing is an indicator of OSA, a common condition with severe health consequences, as discussed throughout this book.

On examination, the base of the tongue was clearly swollen, and was visible in the oropharynx. There was no lymphadenopathy in the neck. She was referred to a head and neck cancer unit for investigation of this gross swelling of the tongue base.

On review in secondary care, the tongue base hypertrophy was visualized on flexible nasendoscopy. There was a very limited oropharyngeal airway. A sleep study demonstrated moderately severe OSA with an AHI of 20.

The oropharynx had the following appearance:

2. What is the next stage for her management?

An unexplained tongue swelling had been identified, and this needed to be addressed on an urgent basis (Figure 34.1). Whilst her symptomatology was not suggestive of cancer, this examination finding was quite suggestive. A biopsy should be undertaken prior to consideration of the management of the sleep disorder.

A large excision of a proportion of the excess tissue was undertaken. The histological diagnosis was lymphoid hyperplasia. This is a rare condition characterized by ongoing proliferation of lymphoid tissue. In this case, lymphoid tissue within the tongue base was leading to upper airway obstruction. Subsequent to the excision, the tissue rapidly recurred.

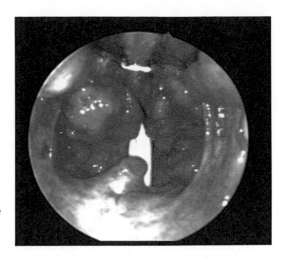

Fig. 34.1 Swelling at the base of the tongue on flexible nasendoscopy examination.

3. What are the options for management of the sleep disorder?

CPAP therapy and MASs are highly unlikely to be successful given the degree and location of the tissue. The two in combination could be considered; however, the extent of the tissue and the rapid recurrence may indicate that the daytime airway may be compromised. The most definitive management option for OSA is tracheostomy insertion. This allows the upper airway to be bypassed completely. In this case, it has the secondary benefit of alleviating any concerns regarding the airway during wakefulness.

The patient underwent semi-elective tracheostomy. This resolved concerns about the airway and improved the sleep quality. However, the patient did have some difficulties acclimatizing to life with a tracheostomy.

4. What tracheostomy care advice should she be given?

A tracheostomy requires close attention to maintain its patency and prevent tracheostomy-associated pneumonia. This includes:

+ regular cleaning
+ regular changing

- ◆ use of an inner cannula
- ◆ suctioning
- ◆ humidification
- ◆ protection when outside.

5. What are the potential complications of tracheostomy?

In the short term, a tracheostomy insertion is associated with risks of infection, bleeding and damage to surrounding structures, including bleeding from the thyroid gland and very rarely paralysis of the vocal cords. Whilst the tracheostomy is in position, the patient may experience swallowing difficulties, and the voice may require the use of particular attachments for the tracheostomy, and may be weaker than it would be otherwise. The long-term complications need to be considered. These range from difficulty in removing the tracheostomy tube (known as decannulation), an increased risk of pneumonia, scarring and fistulation—both tracheo-cutaneous fistulae, and also fistulation into the great vessels, such as tracheo-innominate fistulation. This is a rare, but almost invariably fatal complication. Tracheostomy can lead to tracheal stenosis.

She was able to maintain her tracheostomy care, but found that she had a weak voice with her tracheostomy in situ, and wanted to explore an option to reverse the use of the tracheostomy. Further excision and interstitial radiofrequency thermotherapy in a number of applications over a period of time was used (Figure 34.2).

This was able to control the tongue-base hypertrophy to an extent where it was asymptomatic, although the surgical treatment had to be repeated on a regular basis. A repeat sleep study demonstrated an AHI of 4.

Tracheostomies represent significant undertakings in terms of the effects that they have on a patient's quality of life, and the care they require. Complications are not uncommon and need to be discussed at length prior to proceeding with such a course of treatment. For this reason, tracheostomy is infrequently used for OSA. When it is used, treatment of OSA usually represents just part of the indication. This is the case for this patient, for whom there were concerns about

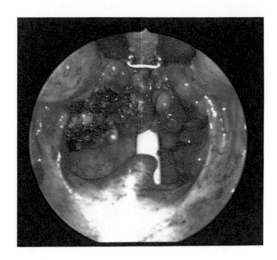

Fig. 34.2 Appearance of swelling at the base of tongue after excision and interstitial radiofrequency thermoplasty.

airway obstruction, and who underwent significant airway surgery. A specific group of patients who undergo tracheostomy partially for the treatment of OSA are paediatric patients with craniosynostosis who, as part of their underlying syndrome, have significant upper airway obstruction during sleep, but also require tracheostomy to facilitate reconstructive craniofacial surgery.

Learning points

Supraglottic and pharyngeal tumours can rarely present with sleep-disordered breathing.

Tracheostomy is a definitive treatment for OSA, but has significant implications for quality of life.

Tracheostomy is most frequently used in the management of OSA in paediatric patients with craniosynostosis or syndromic micrognathia.

Further reading

Cohen SR, Holmes RE, Machado L, Magit A. Surgical strategies in the treatment of complex obstructive sleep apnoea in children. Paediatr Respir Rev 2002 Mar;3(1): 25–35.

Rosen D. Management of obstructive sleep apnea associated with Down's syndrome and other craniofacial dysmorphologies. Curr Opin Pulm Med 2011 Nov;17(6): 431–6.

Section 3

Neurological sleep disorders

Case 35
Sleep groaning

A 23-year-old right-handed woman presented with daytime somnolence and sleepiness for three to four years.

Approximately three to four years ago she was noticed by her then new boyfriend as having episodes at night of holding her breath for approximately 10 seconds, followed by a loud exhaling sound, often resulting in a high-pitched groaning noise. These episodes occurred three to four times a night towards the second half of the night. Her boyfriend would wake her on account of the breath-holding. She does not snore.

There was no past medical history of note. In her family her mother snores, and her grandmother suffers from epilepsy. She sleep-talks at night in full sentences, having conversations with people but making little sense, and there is occasional mumbling.

She goes to bed at about 11 p.m. and sleeps through to 7 a.m.; she is often unrefreshed on waking and will have a one- to two-hour nap early evening after work. On the weekend, she will normally sleep for about twelve hours. She drinks approximately one bottle of wine a week and doesn't smoke.

Neurological examination and examination of the mouth and throat were normal.

Questions

1 What is the cause of the sleep-breathing abnormality and what is the differential diagnosis?
2 How should it be investigated and what will be found?
3 What is the relevance of the sleep-talking?
4 What treatments are appropriate?

Answers

1. What is the cause of the sleep-breathing abnormality and what is the differential diagnosis?

The diagnosis here is catathrenia or sleep groaning. The condition is characterized by breath-holding after inspiration, followed by a groan. Witnesses find both the breath-holding and groan disturbing and will often wake the person. Sleep apnoea is a possible differential, but sleep apnoea results in apnoea spells after expiration and a snorting noise occurs with inspiration. Snoring is also often absent with catathrenia. Another possibility is nocturnal epilepsy. Occasionally, seizures overnight can present with changes in respiration, or groans. In epilepsy, apnoea spells can occur but again usually after expiration; the forced expiration during seizures can result in a groan. However, the description of catathrenia with breath-holding followed by a groan is diagnostic.

2. How should it be investigated and what will be found?

Catathrenia in itself is a benign condition and with a typical history will not need investigation. Reasons for investigating further are an unclear history and/or daytime somnolence, as in this case. The investigation of choice is PSG with respiratory monitoring and a full 10–20 EEG recording. Catathrenia occurs usually during REM sleep and should not be associated with desaturations. In this case, there were frequent episodes of breath-holding during REM sleep lasting

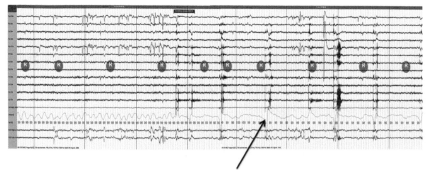

Inspiration followed by slow expiration (groan)

Fig. 35.1 Breathing pattern during REM sleep.

3–20 seconds, sometimes associated with groaning noises with exhalation, typical of catathrenia (Figure 35.1). There were no desaturations or other signs of OSA.

3. What is the relevance of the sleep-talking?
Sleep-talking can occur during all phases of sleep and is very common. It is not specifically associated with catathrenia and it is entirely benign. People rarely say anything of interest in their sleep!

4. What treatments are appropriate?
Treatment of catathrenia is usually unnecessary unless it is waking the person and resulting in daytime somnolence. In my experience, it often responds poorly to medication. However, a sedative such as clonazepam may prevent associated arousals. In severe or distressing cases, CPAP can help.

Learning points

Catathrenia—episodes of breath-holding during inspiration followed by groaning during REM sleep should be differentiated from obstructive apnoea, nocturnal seizures and sleep-talking.

Catathrenia is a benign condition and description of the episodes by a bed partner is diagnostic.

Catathrenia rarely requires treatment—clonazepam helps if the episodes disturb sleep.

Further reading

Iriarte J, Alegre M, Urrestarazu E, Viteri C, Arcocha J, Artieda J. Continuous positive airway pressure as treatment for catathrenia (nocturnal groaning). Neurology 2006;66(4):609–10.

Vetrugno R, Provini F, Plazzi G, Vignatelli L, Lugaresi E, Montagna P. Catathrenia (nocturnal groaning): a new type of parasomnia. Neurology 2001;56(5):681–3.

Case 36
Nocturnal punch and fight

A 75-year-old right-handed man presented with nocturnal episodes over the last 20 years, reported mainly by his wife.

The episodes were occurring almost every night, although he is not aware of many of them. They were worse when he was anxious and have generally become more frequent over the years.

They tend to occur about four to five hours after he has been in bed, and can occur up to four times in a night, but usually just a couple of times. The episodes were described by his wife; he moves from side to side, he can sit up and he can punch out and fight. On occasions he has thrown himself from the bed, and it is on one of these occasions, four years prior, that he sustained an acute subdural, which was evacuated. He does not otherwise usually leave the bed with these episodes. If he wakes from them he will recall a vivid dream during which he is trying to fight against someone or fight someone off. He has no history of sleep-walking. He is an ex-smoker and he does not drink alcohol. There is no family history of note. There was no history of any seizures, meningitis, encephalitis or other parasomnias.

Neurological examination was normal.

Questions

1 What is the diagnosis?

2 With what is this diagnosis associated?

3 What investigations would be recommended?

4 How is this condition best treated?

Answers

1. What is the diagnosis?

The description of the episodes is consistent with an REM sleep behavioural disorder (RBD). This condition is characterized by loss of
normal atonia during REM sleep. During REM sleep, dream enactment occurs, especially enactment of violent or aggressive dreams.
This results in sudden and violent movements that can result in injury
to partner or self. The eyes are usually shut during these episodes and
the person rarely leaves the bed, unless they 'propel' themselves from
the bed. The duration of the movement is usually seconds, but it can
continue for minutes. Episodes of varying intensity will occur most
nights, usually towards the morning (the period when the longest
REM periods occur). RBD is more common in older patients, in particular elderly men.

2. With what is this diagnosis associated?

RBD can be idiopathic and may be familial. In younger people, it is
associated with narcolepsy and can be the presenting symptom of
narcolepsy. In older people, there is a strong association with neurodegenerative disease, in particular Parkinson's disease, multisystem
atrophy and Lewy body dementia (the synucleopathies). However,
other neurodegenerative conditions such as Huntington's disease
and Prion disease can be associated with RBD. The RBD can be the
presenting symptom and can predate other symptoms of neurodegenerative disease by years. With prolonged follow-up, RBD is associated with a neurodegenerative disorder in up to 70% of patients.
DAT (dopamine transporters) scans and tests of olfaction may be
helpful in predicting those who will later develop a synucleopathy.
RBD is also associated with alcohol, recreational drug use and some
medications, including antidepressants.

3. What investigations would be recommended?

PSG is the diagnostic test of choice. Often extra EMG electrodes
(i.e. in addition to the submental EMG) on limbs can help make the
diagnosis. Both loss of normal REM atonia and also an increase in

phasic EMG activity in REM are observed. Investigations for possible causes can be helpful, e.g. the multiple sleep latency test in young people in whom narcolepsy may be suspected, and Dopamine transporter (DaT) and single-photon emission computerized tomography (SPECT) scans and tests of olfaction in the elderly.

4. How is this condition best treated?

Clonazepam is an effective treatment in RBD in suppressing the violent behaviour through suppression of the more violent movements rather than directly restoring the REM atonia. Concerns about tolerance and 'addition' to clonazepam are not usually an issue in RBD. Melatonin is an alternative or adjunctive treatment which may also reduce the loss of REM atonia. Many other treatments have been tried, but there are only small case series or single case reports. In those with Parkinsonism, occasionally increasing the dopaminergic medication can help the RBD. In this case, the RBD responded well to clonazepam 0.5 mg without any increase in dose over the last three years. At his most recent clinic visit, a tremor and some cogwheel rigidity was noted in his right arm, suggestive of early Parkinson's disease.

Learning points

Absence of loss of muscle tone during REM (dream) sleep can lead to dream enactment—REM behavioural disorder (RBD).

RBD may pre-present manifestation of an underlying neurodegenerative disorder.

PSG confirms loss of normal REM sleep atonia.

Further reading

Bonakis A, Howard RS, Ebrahim IO, Merritt S, Williams A. REM sleep behaviour disorder (RBD) and its associations in young patients. Sleep Med 2009;10(6):641–5.

Zanigni S, Calandra-Buonaura G, Grimaldi D, Cortelli P. REM behaviour disorder and neurodegenerative diseases. Sleep Med 2011;12 Suppl 2:S54–8.

Case 37
Jumpy legs

A 39-year-old man presented with worsening daytime somnolence over the last 4 years. He dated his problems to a knee operation, as it was a number of months after this that he would find his overnight sleep unrefreshing. His symptoms have worsened since then and in addition to daytime somnolence, he has had increasing daytime headaches and twitches of his legs and arms when he is tired. He has an ESS score of 18/24 (consistent with excessive daytime somnolence) and he falls asleep most days for usually about half an hour. He goes to bed at 10 p.m. and gets up at 6.45 a.m. unrefreshed. He has jumps of his legs as he goes off to sleep and his partner has noticed large jerks during sleep. He has stopped all caffeinated drinks and rarely drinks alcohol. He gave up tobacco two years ago. He had a septoplasty and interestingly slept better immediately after that when he was taking codeine for the pain.

On direct questioning, he notices that his legs become restless in the evenings and that if he doesn't move them, they can ache—an ache that is relieved by standing up and moving around.

There is no family history of note.

Questions

1 What is the diagnosis?
2 What are the appropriate investigations?
3 How should this be treated and why may his condition have improved after the septoplasty?

Answers

1. What is the diagnosis?

He has periodic limb movement syndrome (PLMS) and restless legs syndrome (RLS). Over 80% of people with RLS also have PLMS, but the converse is not true and only about one-third of people with PLMS have RLS.

RLS is characterized by an overwhelming urge to move the legs and an associated unpleasant sensation in the legs, often described as tingling, cramping or crawling, which gradually worsens if the legs are not moved. These sensations are usually worse in the evening, and movement provides temporary relief. The typical symptoms can be easily remembered using the acronym URGE (Urge to move the legs, Rest worsens, Getting up and moving relieves, Evening preponderance). About 5% of the population is affected by RLS.

RLS needs to be differentiated from cramp (sudden onset of severe pain associated with muscle spasm and relieved with stretching), neuropathy (constant discomfort tingling), vascular insufficiency (worse with movement), arthritis (joint pain) and akathisia (intense restlessness, not usually relieved by movement and associated with neuroleptic use and drug withdrawal).

About 50% of people with RLS have a family history and there are families in which RLS seems to have an autosomal dominant inheritance with anticipation. A number of gene polymorphisms have been associated with RLS, but their role in pathogenesis is unclear. Approximately 40% have an onset before the age of 20 years, and the course tends to be intermittent but progressive. The symptoms can be worsened with stress, concomitant medication (in particular, antidepressant medication) and sleepiness. Sleep disturbance is frequent and often a presenting complaint either due to periodic limb movements or because the RLS prevents the person getting to sleep (insomnia), or on waking in the night, the RLS often prevents the person getting back to sleep. With augmentation and in more severe cases, RLS can also affect the arms and shoulders, and can lose the typical worsening in the evening (occurring occasionally throughout the day).

Periodic limb movements in sleep are brief, repetitive jerks (usually over a period of 0.5–2 seconds but occasionally up to 5 seconds) of usually the legs (arms and trunk can also be affected) that occur usually every 20–40 seconds (this can range from 5–90 seconds). These occur in non-REM sleep and can cause frequent arousals. In contrast to RLS, PLMS are more common in elderly men (>30% of people over the age of 60 years, but fewer than 5% of people under the age of 50 years). PLMS can occur throughout the night in all stages of sleep, but often show a propensity for light sleep, disrupting sleep and preventing the transition to deep sleep. PLMS can therefore present with a history of jerking, but also with daytime somnolence (not all people recognize the jerks). On occasions only the larger jerks are recognized, leading to difficulties in diagnosis, with a differential diagnosis including nocturnal seizures. There is a strong association with not only RLS but also other sleep disorders, including OSA, parasomnia and narcolepsy. Similar to RLS, PLMS can be worsened by sleep deprivation. Both RLS and PLMS can be secondary to peripheral neuropathy (especially diabetic, uraemic and alcoholic neuropathies), iron deficiency, pregnancy and, rarely, spinal cord lesions. There may also be an association with Parkinson's disease.

2. What are the appropriate investigations?

There should be a full neurological examination looking in particular for signs of peripheral neuropathy and extrapyramidal disease. Serum ferritin should be tested. Unless the history is absolutely typical, diagnosis is usually confirmed by PSG with extra EMG electrodes on the limbs. Interestingly, associated sleep disruption is not necessarily correlated with the severity of the movements and in many cases, there is evidence of arousal just prior to the movements, suggesting that the arousal is part of the syndrome rather than merely secondary to the movement. At least four PLMS are required for a diagnosis, and mild, moderate and severe PLMS can be classified as >5, >30 and >50 PLMS per hour overnight.

3. How should this be treated and why may his condition have improved after the septoplasty?

If the serum ferritin is low, then iron should be given. This may help the condition and may also help prevent augmentation if dopamine therapy is used. Good sleep hygiene, prevention of sleep deprivation and avoidance of alcohol and caffeine can all help. Avoidance of certain medication, in particular antidepressants, can also be helpful.

The most effective treatment is a dopamine agonist, and three are licensed for RLS/PLMS—pramipexole, ropinirole and rotigotine patches. L-DOPA can also be used, but has a much greater propensity for augmentation. Augmentation is a worsening of the symptoms while on dopaminergic drugs; this is characterized by earlier onset of symptoms in the day, increased severity, decreased latency and extension of the symptoms to other parts of the body, in particular the arms. In severe cases, jerks can also occur during the day. Increasing the dose of the dopaminergic drug sometimes worsens the augmentation, and alternative therapies are usually needed.

Antiepileptic drugs, in particular pregabalin and gabapentin, but also carbamazepine and valproate, can also be effective. In addition, sedatives such as clonazepam can improve symptoms and in particular can prevent nocturnal arousals, but may have a lesser effect on the motor manifestations.

In more refractory cases and in cases of augmentation, opiates can be used. Codeine is useful in those with milder symptoms, but oxycodone, methadone and fentanyl patches may need to be used in those with more severe symptoms. Sometimes people with RLS/PLMS report improvements in symptoms after operations because of the opiate pain relief (as in this case).

A range of other medication, including baclofen and clonidine, have also been tried and reported in single cases or small case series.

Learning points

Restless legs syndrome is characterized by an uncontrollable urge to move the legs due to an uncomfortable sensation in the legs during the daytime, while PLMS causes sleep disturbance and involuntary kicking of the legs/limbs during sleep. Both conditions often co-exist.

More than four movements during sleep are required for diagnosis of PLMS.

The movements can be controlled by dopamine agonists, antiepileptic drugs or clonazepam.

Further reading

Garcia-Borreguero D, Ferini-Strambi L, Kohnen R, O'Keeffe S, Trenkwalder C, Högl B, Benes H, Jennum P, Partinen M, Fer D, Montagna P, Bassetti CL, Iranzo A, Sonka K, Williams AM. European guidelines on management of restless legs syndrome: report of a joint task force by the European Federation of Neurological Societies, the European Neurological Society and the European Sleep Research Society. Eur J Neurol 2012;19(11):1385–96.

Högl B, Zucconi M, Provini F. RLS, PLM, and their differential diagnosis—a video guide. Mov Disord 2007;22 Suppl 18:S414–19.

Hornyak M, Trenkwalder C, Kohnen R, Scholz H. Efficacy and safety of dopamine agonists in restless legs syndrome. Sleep Med 2012;13(3):228–36.

Satija P, Ondo WG. Restless legs syndrome: pathophysiology, diagnosis and treatment. CNS Drugs 2008;22(6):497–518.

Case 38
Episodic weak legs
in a sleepy man

A 43-year-old man presented with daytime somnolence. He was well until three years ago when he felt exhausted after returning from holiday. He was diagnosed with depression and was started on fluoxetine, but his tiredness continued. About 6 months later, he started to fall asleep during the early evening and then during the day. The episodes were of sudden overwhelming sleepiness and then he would sleep, usually for minutes but sometimes up to an hour. He would be most likely to sleep after lunch or in the early afternoon, or whilst watching TV in the evening. He would dream during this sleep, and would sometime wake, thinking that there was an intruder in his house. On occasions, he has typed nonsense on the computer without realizing that he has done so. His ESS score was 20/24, indicative of excessive daytime somnolence.

He sleeps from 10.30 p.m. until 7 a.m. and does not feel refreshed in the morning. He does not snore excessively and there is no history of periodic limb movements, but there is some history of dream enactment, and he has hit out and shouted in his sleep. He has no hallucinations or vivid dreams as he falls asleep, and the dreams/hallucinations do not occur/continue when he wakes. He has no episodes of paralysis on waking or falling sleep.

Over the last few years, he started reducing his fluoxetine because of weight gain and lack of any benefit. Whilst he was reducing his fluoxetine, he started to have episodes when his legs would buckle, his head would drop and his speech becomes slurred with initially laughter and then subsequently with anger or surprise (such as on unexpectedly seeing a friend). He now has these episodes most days. He could fall, but he holds on to something. These episodes last 15–20 seconds. He does not smoke and drinks about 14–21 units per week. There is no family history of note.

Questions

1 What condition does he have, what features does he have and what does he lack?

2 What investigations would be helpful?

3 What neurological conditions are associated?

4 What treatments are appropriate?

Answers

1. What condition does he have, what features does he have and what does he lack?

His symptoms are consistent with a diagnosis of narcolepsy, which has a prevalence of about 1 in 2,000 people. The presenting symptoms are usually excessive daytime somnolence with irresistible sleep attacks during the day, often occurring at inappropriate time, and often associated with dreaming. He also has cataplexy, which was probably initially masked by the antidepressant medication fluoxetine. Cataplexy is the occurrence of brief episodes of loss of muscle power/tone that is precipitated by strong emotion, such as laughter, anger or surprise (unexpectedly seeing a familiar person can precipitate an attack). Mild attacks usually consist of transient drooping of the eyelids, mouth and head, and there is often slurred speech. The tone can return in an intermittent fashion, giving the impression of head and mouth jerking. In more severe forms the limbs are affected, leading in some instances to collapse. Cataplexy usually lasts for a brief period (seconds or minutes) and may be followed by a sleep episode. Over 70% of people with narcolepsy have cataplexy and it usually occurs after the excessive daytime somnolence, but on occasions may predate the somnolence. Other typical symptoms are sleep paralysis, and hypnogogic (on falling asleep) and hypnopompic (on waking) hallucinations, which he does not have. These are symptoms that can commonly occur in people without narcolepsy and so are not particularly specific. Other typical features that he has are a disrupted night's sleep and short periods of automatic behaviour during the daytime (micro-sleeps). It is important to realize that narcolepsy is an abnormality of sleep regulation rather than the amount of sleep someone requires, and so despite the daytime somnolence, nocturnal sleep is often disturbed and disrupted (some even complain of insomnia). Lastly, REM behavioural disorder is common in narcolepsy (loss of REM atonia is seen in most people with narcolepsy with cataplexy) and on occasions can be the presenting symptom.

2. What investigations would be helpful?

PSG and multiple sleep latency tests should be performed in most people with narcolepsy. PSG is important to exclude other possible causes of somnolence including OSA, period limb movements of sleep and REM-related behaviour disorder, especially because these are all more common in people with narcolepsy. PSG may also demonstrate early onset sleep (within 10 minutes) and early onset REM (within 20 minutes). The multiple sleep latency test (MSLT) is used to confirm the diagnosis. In this test the patient is allowed to fall asleep four to five times at two-hourly intervals throughout the day and the latency to sleep onset is measured. People are permitted to sleep for 15 minutes and a sleep onset REM is defined as an REM period occurring within this time. Most diagnostic criteria require, as a minimum, a mean sleep latency on MSLT of ≤ eight minutes and two or more sleep onset REM periods following at least six hours of nocturnal sleep during the night prior to the test.

There is a strong correlation between narcolepsy (with cataplexy) and HLA type. Indeed, in contrast to dogs, in which narcolepsy is related to mutations in the hypocretin (orexin) receptors, narcolepsy in humans is usually an autoimmune condition and recently antibodies to a specific protein expressed in the hypothalamus, Trib2, have been described in people with narcolepsy. Of the HLA alleles, the HLA-DQB1*06:02 subtype is strongly (~90%) associated with narcolepsy with cataplexy (less strongly associated if cataplexy is not present). However, this subtype is very common (20–30%) in the general population and therefore the positive predictive value is low, and so this test has limited diagnostic use. Measurement of CSF hypocretin (orexin) levels can be useful in those with cataplexy in whom the levels are less than 110 ng/L, or one-third of the mean control values. However, its use in those without cataplexy is unclear, and when a definite diagnosis of cataplexy is present, especially in combination with other typical symptoms and a diagnostic MSLT, it is difficult to see how this test adds much to the diagnosis.

Other tests such as MRI scan in those without other neurological symptoms have a very low yield.

3. What neurological conditions are associated?

Most cases of narcolepsy are idiopathic. However, there are cases of symptomatic narcolepsy associated with brain lesions in the third ventricle/hypothalamus. These include vascular lesions, tumours, demyelination and encephalitis. Other neurological signs (in particular, brain stem signs) are almost always present in such cases. In addition, narcolepsy can be associated with head trauma, although the presence of a causal lesion in such cases is not always apparent. Narcolepsy with cataplexy has also been associated with Niemann–Pick disease (a metabolic disorder resulting in sphingomyelin accumulation in the brain, liver and spleen) or Prader–Willi syndrome (a chromosomal disorder affecting chromosome 15). Isolated cataplexy has also been associated with such lesions, as well as with inherited conditions such as Norrie disease (an X-linked disorder with blindness, deafness, learning difficulties and dysmorphic features), Coffin Lowry syndrome (an X-linked disorder with severe learning difficulties, dysmorphism and skeletal abnormalities including kyphoscoliosis) and Möbius syndrome (congenital facial and abducens nerve palsies).

4. What treatments are appropriate?

Non-pharmacological approaches to treatment include good sleep hygiene and planned daytime naps. The preferred treatment for EDS is modafinil, which does not usually result in tolerance and has fewer peripheral side effects compared to the amphetamines. Alternatives are amphetamines, including dexamphetamine and methylphenidate. These can be associated with hypertension and tolerance. However in contrast to modafinil, the amphetamines may also help cataplexy.

Cataplexy can often resolve with an improvement in nocturnal sleep and daytime somnolence, and also often improve with age. The mainstay of treatment is antidepressant drugs including clomipramine, fluoxetine and venlafaxine. These are also effective against other REM-related symptoms. More recently, the sedative sodium oxybate has been shown to be effective against all narcolepsy symptoms, but its use has been largely restricted by price.

Other associated sleep disorders including poor nocturnal sleep, periodic limb movements and sleep apnoea may require treatment and if present, may make daytime somnolence more difficult to treat.

Learning points

Classical narcolepsy tetrad consists of daytime sleepiness, cataplexy, sleep paralysis and hypnogogic hallucinations.

Sleep onset REM sleep on PSG and reduced sleep latency <8 minutes on multiple sleep latency test is required for confirmation of diagnosis.

It is idiopathic in most patients and HLA linked—thought to be due to autoimmune damage to hypothalamus.

Pharmacological approach is helpful in controlling symptoms.

Further reading

Billiard M, Bassetti C, Dauvilliers Y, Dolenc-Groselj L, Lammers GJ, Mayer G, Pollmächer T, Reading P, Sonka K. EFNS Task Force. EFNS guidelines on management of narcolepsy. Eur J Neurol 2006;13(10):1035–48.

Cvetkovic-Lopes V, Bayer L, Dorsaz S, Maret S, Pradervand S, Dauvilliers Y, Lecendreux M, Lammers GJ, Donjacour CE, Du Pasquier RA, Pfister C, Petit B, Hor H, Mühlethaler M, Tafti M. Elevated Tribbles homolog 2-specific antibody levels in narcolepsy patients. J Clin Invest 2010;120(3):713–19.

Dauvilliers Y, Billiard M, Montplaisir J. Clinical aspects and pathophysiology of narcolepsy. Clin Neurophysiol 2003;114(11):2000–17.

Keam S, Walker MC. Therapies for narcolepsy with or without cataplexy: evidence-based review. Curr Opin Neurol 2007;20(6):699–703.

Case 39
Just sleepy all the time

A 47-year-old woman presented with EDS. She is only awake for about 4–6 hours a day; the rest of the time she spends in bed sleeping. She can date her sleepiness back to her twenties, but is unaware of any precipitating event. Her sleepiness worsened over a few years but has remained much unchanged over the last 20 years. She describes an urge to sleep for most of the day. However, she has not fallen asleep in strange situations and is able to remain awake when required. She has an ESS score of 20/24. She goes to bed at 8 p.m. and sleeps through to 10–11 a.m. She will sleep through alarm clocks and has in the past used three or four alarm clocks to wake her. Apparently, she sleeps like a 'log' and there is no history of leg movements or snoring. When she gets up, she feels quite unsteady and muzzy-headed, and has fallen on occasions. She will fall asleep during the day sometimes for hours, and on waking she will feel unrefreshed. She does not recall any dreams. There is no history of hypnogogic or hypnopompic hallucinations or sleep paralysis. There is no history of sudden weakness or head drops with laughter or strong emotion.

She was diagnosed with depression in the past, and has been treated with a variety of antidepressants without any benefit.

She has one daughter aged 28 years old who is well, but she is a long sleeper, usually requiring 10–12 hours sleep at night.

Neurological examination was unremarkable.

Questions

1 What is the diagnosis and why is she unsteady in the morning?
2 What would you expect PSG and multiple sleep latency tests to show?
3 What would be the appropriate treatments?

Answers

1. What is the diagnosis and why is she unsteady in the morning?

The diagnosis here is idiopathic hypersomnia, which is a rare disorder characterized by excessive daytime somnolence but without cataplexy, usually starting in adolescence. The daytime sleeps are usually resistible, long (often over an hour), unrefreshing and not associated with REM phenomena. Idiopathic hypersomnia is a heterogeneous disorder and can be associated with normal overnight sleep or with prolonged nocturnal sleep times (>10 hours in bed) in which the person often sleeps through alarm clocks. The differential diagnosis includes narcolepsy (see Table 39.1) and other disorders that can disrupt nocturnal sleep, such as periodic limb movements of sleep and sleep apnoea. However, the main differential diagnosis is behaviourally induced insufficient sleep syndrome, in which the person (sometimes unwittingly) is getting insufficient sleep at night (actigraphy and, occasionally, sleep diaries can help in the differential diagnosis). The morning symptoms here of 'sleep drunkenness' are common and characterized by disorientation, confusion, slowed cognition, unsteadiness and sleepiness.

Table 39.1 Features that distinguish narcolepsy from idiopathic hypersomnia

Feature	Sensitivity (%)	Specificity (%)
Sleep drunkenness	55	97
MSLT ≥8 minutes	49	93
Night sleep ≥9 hours	58	92
Nap ≥60 minutes	87	87
Absence of vivid dreams	75	81
Sleep efficiency ≥90%	84	65
REM latency ≥50 minutes	94	48

2. What would you expect PSG and multiple sleep latency tests to show?

The PSG often shows shortened sleep latency, increased TST (often increased deep sleep) and normal REM sleep onset. The multiple sleep latency test demonstrates fewer than two sleep onset REMs. The latency is variable, and those with prolonged nocturnal sleep may in many cases be within normal limits. However, in those with a normal sleep time, many would require a latency of less than 8 minutes to be necessary for diagnosis. Actinography in those with prolonged sleep shows >10 hours sleep per day.

CSF hypocretin (orexin) tends not to be useful for diagnosis, as it is usually low or normal.

3. What would be the appropriate treatments?

Stimulants are helpful and are similar to those used in narcolepsy (e.g. modafinil, dexamfetamine and methylphenidate). Caffeine can also be helpful and many patients describe that a morning coffee helps with the sleep drunkenness. In those with long sleep times and difficulty getting up in the morning, modafinil at bedtime can be helpful.

Learning points

Idiopathic hypersomnia is a rare cause of marked daytime sleepiness, but other common causes should be excluded first.

It can be difficult to distinguish from narcolepsy, but PSG can help.

Stimulants can help to reduce daytime sleepiness.

Further reading

Anderson KN, Pilsworth S, Sharples LD, Smith IE, Shneerson JM. Idiopathic hypersomnia: a study of 77 cases. Sleep 2007 Oct;30(10):1274–81.

2. What would you expect PSG and multiple sleep latency tests to show?

The PSG often shows shortened sleep latency, increased TST (often increased deep sleep) and normal REM sleep pattern. The multiple sleep latency test demonstrates lower than average sleep REMs. The latency is variable, and those with profound/abnormal sleep in these cases is lower than normal. This is because both sleep latency and REM sleep onset latency are lower.

Case 40
Moving and thrashing around during sleep

A 32-year-old man presented with restless and broken sleep since around the age of 16 years. His mother mentioned that he has always been active in his sleep, moving about and thrashing around. There is also a possible history of some sleepwalking in his teens, although this no longer occurs. He usually goes to bed around 11 p.m.–12.30 a.m. at night, and gets up at 6.30 a.m. during the week and at 7.30 a.m. at weekends.

He does not feel refreshed. He is aware of waking a couple of times at night. His wife reports that he is restless in his sleep and there may be some kicking movements. There is also a history of mild snoring, but his wife also noted that there were episodes of heavy breathing rather than snoring and this appears in episodes during the night but not every night.

Although he is tired during the day, his ESS score was only 8/24. He keeps active during the day to avoid falling asleep. If he does permit himself to take a nap, usually for 20–30 minutes, he feels more refreshed.

There is no history of any sleep paralysis or any visual hallucinations. There is no history of any cataplexy, but sometimes when he is very tired he feels his muscles are weak, and when he laughs a lot his legs feel weak. There is no antecedent history of note. His father had a history of depression and insomnia, but there was no other history of note.

He lives with his wife. He works as a van driver and he takes a nap prior to driving if he has to travel long distances. He does not smoke or drink alcohol. He had been investigated with an MRI and a daytime EEG, which were normal.

In view of his sleepiness, he was admitted for PSG and a multiple sleep latency test. During the PSG, he was noted to have eight stereotypical events arising from both light and deep sleep in which he suddenly appears to rouse, and then both arms stiffen and he makes cycling movements with his legs for about 10 seconds. The EEG during these events is obscured by artefact. Otherwise, the EEG only shows some bursts of non-specific slow waves over the frontal regions. The multiple sleep latency test revealed a mean sleep latency of 12 minutes with no sleep onset REM.

Questions

1 What is the likely diagnosis here?
2 What is the appropriate treatment?
3 What should he do about his driving?

Answers

1. What is the likely diagnosis here?

The most likely diagnosis of stereotypical, brief events occurring many times at night during both light and deep sleep (but rarely from REM sleep) is nocturnal epilepsy. Approximately 20% of people with epilepsy have predominantly nocturnal seizures and 6% have exclusively nocturnal seizures. Sudden drug withdrawal or frequent seizures increase the risk of daytime seizures. Nocturnal tonic–clonic seizures are usually easy to diagnose in those who share a bed, but can be difficult in those who sleep alone; clues may include nocturnal incontinence (also caused by enuresis), tongue biting (also caused by facio-mandibular myoclonus), muscle aches and morning headaches. The other common nocturnal seizures are nocturnal frontal lobe seizures. Nocturnal frontal lobe seizures can manifest as (i) paroxysmal arousals, which consist of brief, sudden eye opening, head raising or sitting up in bed, a frightened expression and, sometimes, vocalization or nocturnal paroxysmal dystonia, which involves dystonic posturing, and (ii) hypermotor phenomena such as kicking, running or cycling movements of the legs. Episodic nocturnal wanderings have also been described, but in many cases these may be a parasomnia precipitated by the seizure. Daytime interictal EEG shows epileptiform abnormalities in up to one-third of cases; this increases to 50% with nocturnal EEGs. Ictal EEG is often unhelpful, as it is often obscured by artefact.

It is essential to distinguish epilepsy from non-REM parasomnia and REM behavioural disorder, and the frontal lobe epilepsy and parasomnias (FLEP) scale can be helpful (see Table 40.1).

In cases where there is doubt about the diagnosis, video-EEG telemetry is necessary. On occasions, people may be unaware of the seizures and present solely with daytime somnolence. On occasions, nocturnal frontal lobe epilepsy can be inherited as an autosomal dominant condition and has been associated with mutation in the nicotinic acetylcholine receptor.

Table 40.1 FLEP score. Total ≤0 is indicative of parasomnia and >3 is indicative of epilepsy

Feature	Score
Age of onset ≥55y	−1
Duration <2 mins	+1
Duration >10 mins	−2
Typically 3–5 in a night	+1
Typically >5 in a night	+2
Occur <30 mins of sleep	+1
Definite aura	+2
Wandering outside bedroom	−2
Complex directed behaviour	−2
Prominent dystonic posturing	+1
Highly stereotypical	+1
Highly variable	−1
Lucid recall	+1
Coherent speech with poor/no recall	−2
Coherent speech with recall	+2
TOTAL	

2. What is the appropriate treatment?

No treatment is an option, but nocturnal seizures are associated with sudden unexplained death in epilepsy, and also in this case he feels tired during the day. The favoured treatments in focal epilepsy are lamotrigine and carbamazepine (carbamazepine seems to be particularly effective in the autosomal dominant nocturnal frontal lobe epilepsies). Also, people with autosomal dominant nocturnal frontal lobe epilepsies find that nicotine can help and there is anecdotal evidence that in these patients nicotine patches can be helpful.

3. What should he do about his driving?

The driving regulations in UK for epilepsy are clear insofar as:

If the person has only had sleep seizures and this pattern has been established for one year, then they can drive. If they have also had seizures when awake, then they can drive once the pattern of solely sleep seizures has been established for three years.

Therefore, in this case, the seizures (which have been present for many years) will not prevent the patient from driving. He will, however, have to inform the DVLA. The rules about sleepiness are less clear and people should not drive if they are sleepy.

Learning points

Sleep disruption due to nocturnal epilepsy should be distinguished from REM behavioural disorders and non-REM parasomnias.

The FLEP scale can help to distinguish between the two conditions.

Further reading

Derry CP, Davey M, Johns M, Kron K, Glencross D, Marini C, Scheffer IE, Berkovic SF. Distinguishing sleep disorders from seizures: diagnosing bumps in the night. Arch Neurol 2006;63(5):705–9.

Provini F, Plazzi G, Tinuper P, Vandi S, Lugaresi E, Montagna P. Nocturnal frontal lobe epilepsy. A clinical and polygraphic overview of 100 consecutive cases. Brain 1999;122 (Pt6):1017–31.

Case 41
Panic attacks during sleep

A 50-year-old man presented with nocturnal events going back at least to the age of 19 years. They were now occurring two to three times per month. His wife had witnessed quite a number of these events. The events had some stereotypical features; whilst sleeping, he would suddenly sit up on the bed and shout, 'No, no, no'. He would look very panicky and frightened, and appeared confused. He would then walk around the room, get back into bed and go back to sleep within about ten minutes. The events occurred sometimes up to four times at night, but usually once or twice. They did not have any particular temporal pattern during the night, but occurred at least an hour after sleep. There was no family history of note and the neurological examination was normal.

These episodes had been diagnosed as seizures because of their stereotypy and he was prescribed carbamazepine, which he took, but it had no beneficial effect and made him drowsy, so he stopped the medication.

Questions

1 What is the differential diagnosis for these events?
2 How does the temporal pattern and number of events help?
3 If the events had improved with carbamazepine, would this have helped the diagnosis?
4 What tests would be appropriate?

to identify these, and treatment of these conditions can lead to a resolution of the non-REM parasomnia.

Learning points

Apparent panic attacks during sleep can be due to nocturnal epilepsy or non-REM parasomnia.

In non-REM parasomnia, the frontal brain area sleeps whilst the limbic system wakes.

It can be treated with long-acting benzodiazepines.

Further reading

Derry CP, Harvey AS, Walker MC, Duncan JS, Berkovic SF. NREM arousal parasomnias and their distinction from nocturnal frontal lobe epilepsy: a video EEG analysis. Sleep 2009;32(12):1637–44.

Case 42
Frozen in sleep

A 38-year-old woman presented with a history of being unable to move on waking since her teenage years. This can occur just as she is going to sleep or she can wake in the night with the sensation. She feels unable to move and sometimes, especially in the past, she felt as if she had trouble breathing. On rare occasions, she has felt as if there is someone present, sometimes pressing down on her chest. In the past, she would panic, which seemed to prolong the episode. More recently, the episodes have been briefer and she seems to snap out of them. Often, if she can concentrate on moving a finger or toe, this can end the episode. She can have weeks between episodes, but in recent months, following a change in her job, she is having episodes every night. She thinks her mother may have had similar episodes, but her mother is no longer living and she has a teenage daughter who has started to complain of similar episodes, although occurring infrequently.

Questions

1 What is this condition and with what is it associated?
2 What investigations would you arrange?
3 How is this best treated?

Answers

1. What is this likely to be and what other symptoms would you ask about?

This is a recurrent hypersomnia and the symptoms are consistent with Kleine–Levin syndrome. This condition usually occurs in adolescents and in males, but can occur throughout adult life. It is rare, with a prevalence of approximately two to ten per million. Many people describe an infection as a precipitant, but no infectious or autoimmune cause has been found. The typical symptoms during episodes, which last days to weeks, that occur in addition to the somnolence are detailed in Table 43.1. In addition to the cognitive problems, irritability and autonomic symptoms that occurred in this man, abnormal eating behaviour, in particular megaphagia, often occurs. Hypersexuality during episodes also occasionally occurs.

2. What is the prognosis and what treatments would you suggest?

Although people are said to be normal between episodes, it is the experience of these authors that the disruptive nature of the episodes can often have a profound psychosocial effect on people with this condition, so that they can become depressed and socially withdrawn. The condition resolves within about ten years in approximately half the people who have it. Ranges of medication have been

Table 43.1 Symptoms

Symptoms	Incidence
Cognitive disorder	96%
(abnormal speech, confusion, amnesia, derealization, hallucinations, delusions)	
Eating behaviour disorder	80%
(megaphagia, craving for sweets)	
Irritability	92%
Hypersexuality	43%
Depression	48%

used to prevent attacks including lithium, antiepileptic drugs and antidepressants. Treatment with stimulants during the episodes can be helpful, but are often poorly tolerated.

Learning points

Episodes of sleepiness, associated with cognitive problems, and irritability in a young person can be due to a rare disorder called Kleine–Levin syndrome.

It either resolves spontaneously or can be controlled with medications.

Further reading

Arnulf I, Rico TJ, Mignot E. Diagnosis, disease course, and management of patients with Kleine–Levin syndrome. Lancet Neurol 2012 Oct;11(10):918–28.

Arnulf I, Zeitzer JM, File J, Farber N, Mignot E. Kleine–Levin syndrome: a systematic review of 186 cases in the literature. Brain 2005;128(Pt 12):2763–76.

Case 44
Chattering teeth during sleep

A 56-year-old man presented with repeated episodes of tongue biting at night. This had occurred over the last year about eight times, and on several occasions he had found blood on his pillow. He had usually bitten the side of his tongue and it would be sore for a day or so. The tongue biting had not woken him, and when he woke in the morning there were no other symptoms, in particular no muscle aches and no incontinence. He shared a bed with his wife and she had not noticed any abnormal movements or convulsions, but reported that her husband's teeth sometimes made a chattering noise at night. There was no prior history of epilepsy, and no antecedent history of note. There was no family history of epilepsy or any sleep disorder. He had had an MRI brain scan which was normal, and a daytime EEG which was within normal limits.

Questions

1 What is the differential diagnosis and what is the likely diagnosis here?

2 What are the treatment options?

Answers

1. What is the differential diagnosis and what is the likely diagnosis here?

Tongue biting at night can be indicative of seizures, facio-mandibular myoclonus and bruxism. Seizures usually result in other signs (e.g. convulsion) that would be apparent to a bed partner. When a bed partner is not present, the differential diagnosis can be more challenging; seizures, however, are often associated with other symptoms in the morning, including muscle aches, muzzy-headedness and headache. It is rare with bruxism to draw blood, and usually the cheek rather than the tongue is chewed. Facio-mandibular myoclonus is a benign condition characterized by jerking of the mouth and jaw (masticatory muscles), usually during REM sleep, and can commonly result in tongue biting (often the side of the tongue is bitten, as occurs in seizures). Blood can be drawn and the person may not wake with the tongue biting, leading to diagnostic difficulties. Bed partners can report a tapping or clicking of the teeth, as in the case here.

2. What are the treatment options?

The best treatment for this condition is unclear. Clonazepam has been reported to be helpful. In contrast to bruxism, there is not necessarily any grinding of the teeth and so a splint is unnecessary.

Learning points

Tongue biting and a chattering noise during sleep could be due to facio-mandibular myoclonus and responds well to clonazepam.

Bruxism—teeth grinding does not cause tongue biting.

Further reading

Seneviratne U. Facio-mandibular myoclonus: a rare cause of nocturnal tongue biting. Epileptic Disord 2011;13(1):96–8.

Case 45
Sexsomnia

A 23-year-old man presented with episodes of sex during his sleep. From about the age of 6 years, he talked in his sleep and would occasionally shout out and run into his parents' room, where he would be quite confused. He would have no recollection of these episodes in the morning. These episodes continued into adulthood. On occasions, he would report a dream as if he was being chased and struggling to run. These events would occur in the middle of the night. In addition, usually one to three hours after he had gone to sleep, he would sit up suddenly, look scared and not respond appropriately. He usually went back to sleep after this and would often be amnesic for these events. He would usually sleep for eight hours at night, but had broken, disturbed sleep. In the last two to three years he had started to have sex with his partner in the middle of the night and he would have no recollection of doing so. His partner described the intercourse as often unwanted and it would be rougher than normal, without any foreplay. On occasion, she could push him off and he would appear confused or incompletely responsive. These episodes were having an impact on their relationship.

Other than a past history of depression, there had been no past history of note.

There is a strong family history of walking and talking in sleep, including his maternal grandfather and his mother.

Neurological examination was normal.

Question

1 What is the diagnosis here?

Answer

1. What is the diagnosis here?

This man has a non-REM parasomnia, and the sexual acts are likely to be sexsomnia (a form of non-REM parasomnia). Although the commonest forms of non-REM parasomnia are sleepwalking, night terrors and confusional arousals, more elaborate behaviour such as sleep-eating and sexsomnia can occur in adults. Non-REM parasomnias usually occur from slow-wave (deep) sleep, within two to three hours of falling asleep. They are commoner in children (affecting 20–30%) and usually resolve by adolescence. However, it has been estimated that over 5% of adults have non-REM parasomnia (usually sleepwalking or night terrors). There is usually a family history of non-REM parasomnias.

Non-REM parasomnia can be triggered by sleep deprivation and stress; the role of alcohol is less certain. People are invariably unaware during the event, and are often totally amnesic for the event. There is no specific diagnostic test for non-REM parasomnia, other than recording them with video and EEG (to confirm the stage of sleep in which they occur).

The repertoire of sexual behaviours that can occur during non-REM parasomnia (sexsomnia) includes masturbation, sexual fondling, oral sex and vaginal or anal intercourse. Sexsomnia has been described more frequently in men than women. Reported triggers for sexsomnia include physical contact with another person in bed, alcohol, fatigue, stress, sleep deprivation and drug abuse.

Learning points

Non-REM parasomnias can cause physical sexual acts during sleep, in addition to sleep talking, walking and eating.

Further reading

Schenck CH, Arnulf I, Mahowald MW. Sleep and sex: what can go wrong? A review of the literature on sleep related disorders and abnormal sexual behaviors and experiences. Sleep 2007 Jun;30(6):683–702.

Section 4

Insomnia and circadian rhythm disorders

Case 46
I keep falling asleep at family dinners

Mr D is a retired civil servant with acquired retinal blindness who presented to the insomnia clinic with a complaint of waking too early in the morning. He was waking at around 4 a.m. every day and, while this in itself was not troubling him, the early start meant he was feeling sleepy early in the evenings. He would often nod off at family dinners and would generally be in bed asleep by 9 p.m. at the latest. He found this extremely frustrating while he was working, but it did not interfere with his occupational functioning. However, when he retired he resolved to indulge his passion for theatre and opera, but he kept falling asleep in the theatres and missing the performances. This motivated him to address the issue.

Mr D said he had always been an early riser and did his best work in the morning. He had always gone to bed earlier than his wife, but his cycle had gradually shifted forward as he got older. When he woke at 4 a.m.–5 a.m. he would immediately feel alert and be unable to go back to sleep no matter how long he stayed in bed. He therefore usually got up immediately on waking in the morning. He generally felt well and alert throughout the day, but started to feel sleepy at around 7 p.m.

Questions

1 What is the most likely diagnosis?
2 How would you confirm the diagnosis?
3 How would you treat this?

Answers

1. What is the most likely diagnosis?

Mr D is most likely suffering from an advanced sleep phase syndrome (ASPS). His circadian rhythm is 24 hours long, but his body clock is advanced relative to the outside world. ASPS is the opposite of a delayed sleep phase syndrome (DSPS) and is less common. It may be under-reported to some extent, as it causes less occupational dysfunction. Whereas DSPS patients have difficulty getting up in time for work, are often sleepy deprived and are very sleep in the mornings, ASPS patients are able to get to work on time and, as they are usually able to go to bed early in the evening, are less likely to be sleep deprived. Furthermore, society tends to approve of this 'early to bed, early to rise' lifestyle, but late to bed and late to rise is discouraged. However, the difficulty in staying awake in the evenings does have a negative impact on the patient, particularly with regard to their social life.

2. How would you confirm the diagnosis?

The diagnosis of ASPS is generally made on history and investigations rarely add much value. A sleep diary is often helpful in terms of getting a longitudinal picture of the sleep cycle. Patients will often describe either their most recent night or their worst night, and so having a couple of weeks of a sleep diary allows you to get a fuller picture. It will also allow you to see if the sleep complaint is constant, how much night-to-night variability there is and how often the patient is using medication, alcohol, etc. to manage their condition.

If objective evidence of their sleep pattern is required, one can perform actigraphy. The patient wears an actigraph (a wristwatch-like apparatus with a small accelerometer) on their wrist, usually for one to three weeks. The actigraph measures their movement and this information can be used to determine when the person is awake and asleep. In ASPS one would expect to see early sleep onset and early awakening.

One can also perform an objective measure of the patient's melatonin rhythm with a dim light melatonin onset (DLMO) test. In this test the patient provides serial saliva samples whilst in a dimly lit room and these samples are then analysed to determine the melatonin level. In a normal subject one would expect to see a fairly abrupt rise in melatonin levels around 9 p.m. In patients with ASPS this would occur earlier, while in patients with DSPS it would occur later. In fact, the DLMO test is very rarely done in clinical settings and is largely used as a research tool. However, it can be useful for determining the optimum timing of melatonin and light treatment, as well as in cases where there is a suspicion that the shift in sleep cycle may be due to lifestyle factors rather than a circadian rhythm disorder.

Mr D kept a sleep diary for two weeks, and the second week is reproduced in Table 46.1

The diary confirmed a consistent early sleep onset time and wake time. As you can see, he also fell asleep before going to bed on three nights, including at the dinner table during a family birthday celebration.

3. How would you treat this?

The strongest evidence base for the treatment of ASPS is using bright light in the evening to delay the person's sleep phase. This should ideally be coupled with avoidance of light in the early part of the morning. However, positive studies have typically used high doses for extended periods and compliance with this regime can be difficult. Use of natural daylight when possible is preferred; otherwise a seasonal affective disorder (SAD) lamp can be used. Obviously, in Mr D's case, light is not going to be helpful, as he is completely blind.

Taking melatonin in the second half of the sleep period, or immediately on waking, would in theory delay the patient's phase. However, there is no trial data to support this practice. The other factor to consider is that melatonin, in addition to having a circadian rhythm shifting effect, is also mildly sedative. There are therefore legitimate concerns that taking melatonin in the second half of the night might

Table 46.1 Sleep diary of a patient with ASPS

Week starting: 01.07.11	Last night I went to bed at:	This morning I got up at:	So I was in bed for (hr:min):	It took me ? minutes to fall asleep:	I woke ? number of times:	During the night I was awake for:	In total I think I slept for:	Other info:
Night 1	20:30	05:00	8:30	5	1	5	8:10	2 glasses of wine
Night 2	20:00	05:15	9:15	2	1	5	9:00	
Night 3	22:45	05:00	6:15	2	1	5	6:10	Fell asleep at opera!
Night 4	20:00	04:15	8:15	5	1	5	8:05	Fell asleep at dinner!
Night 5	20:40	04:50	8:10	0	2	15	7:55	
Night 6	20:05	05:00	8:55	10	1	5	8:40	Fell asleep in front of TV
Night 7	20:50	06:00	9:10	2	1	55	8:15	Had lie-in, but no extra sleep
Average in hours and minutes	20:41	05:02	8:21	3.7	1.1	13.6	8:02	

lead to excessive daytime sedation, particularly in drivers. Further, there is very little evidence regarding the efficacy of stimulants and hypnotics in these patients. Using a very short-acting hypnotic, such as zaleplon, on waking would probably extend the sleep period, but would not impact on the underlying circadian rhythm disorder. Stimulants in the evening to help patients stay awake have been used in individual patients with some success.

Our initial strategy with Mr D was to institute behavioural interventions. As we could not use light, we needed to find other wakefulness-promoting stimuli to try to keep him awake later in the evening. We therefore encouraged him to engage in physical exercise in the evening and he arranged for his family to take him for a brisk walk outdoors every evening before dinner. He found that this helped him stay awake during dinner and delayed his sleep onset, but only by about 30 minutes, and he was still waking up early in the morning. He had previously tried using caffeine to keep himself awake at night, but found it not particularly effective. However, it seemed to be slightly more effective when combined with the physical exercise.

Mr D decided that he would like to have a trial of melatonin and so we prescribed 2 mg slow-release melatonin (the only licensed preparation in the United Kingdom). He was concerned about the risk of daytime sedation and so he decided to cut the pills into quarters using a pill cutter. As you can see from his diary, he wakes at least once a night, usually to pass water, and the waking time was very consistent. He would generally wake between 2.30 and 3.00 a.m., and we felt this was a good time to take the melatonin.

He therefore woke, went to the toilet to pass water, took the melatonin and then went back to sleep almost immediately. Within a week his circadian rhythm shifted and he was falling asleep around 11.00 p.m., was still waking to pass water around 2.30–3.00 a.m. and was then sleeping through to 7.00 a.m. He was not experiencing any side effects from the medication and was much more alert in the evenings. The improvement was maintained at follow-up 1 year later.

Answers

1. What is sleep hygiene and how does it work?

Sleep hygiene is a term used to describe the common-sense lifestyle factors that are thought to affect sleep. It includes things such as avoiding all caffeine after 4 p.m., taking exercise, having a warm bath in the evening, ensuring the room is dark and quiet, etc. It is probably the most widely distributed advice to insomnia patients, but actually the evidence is that when taken on its own it does not work! In fact, the results of sleep hygiene interventions are so disappointing that it is often used as the placebo in insomnia treatment studies. There is insufficient evidence to say with any certainty whether it confers any benefit when combined with other techniques. Despite this, it is routinely included in cognitive behaviour therapy (CBT) for insomnia treatment programmes. To some extent this is because sleep hygiene is so entrenched in the insomnia treatment culture that it is almost expected as part of any treatment package. It is also thought that if patients get their sleep hygiene very wrong, it will make it harder for the effective techniques to work. Finally, anecdotally some patients do derive benefit from the sleep hygiene advice.

Mrs W followed the sleep hygiene rules strictly, cutting out all caffeine after lunch, avoiding alcohol, walking 6 km every morning, having a warm bath every night and meditating for 10 minutes before going to bed. She found it made no difference whatsoever, which further strengthened her conviction that her insomnia was not due to lifestyle or psychological factors, but was rather due to an underlying organic disorder.

She returned to the GP insisting that he prescribe hypnotics. She had by now stopped breastfeeding, but the GP was concerned that she still needed to be alert enough to attend to her children at night. He therefore prescribed 10 mg of Amitriptyline, but Mrs W said this did not improve her sleep at all and it made her feel 'like a zombie' the next day. This is unfortunately a common side effect of the sedative antidepressants, which tend to have a long half-life and therefore lead to significant daytime sedation. Her husband, who had been working on an oil rig, left his job and moved into a nine-to-five office-based job so he could help his wife cope and spend more time with the children. Now that he was going to be home at night, the GP agreed to prescribe hypnotics. He tried temazepam, zopiclone and zolpidem, but Mrs W insisted that she didn't sleep at all on these pills, even when she took three or four at a time. This raised her anxiety further and she demanded to be referred to a sleep clinic. The GP made the referral but it was rejected, as the local sleep clinics did not treat insomnia.

Mrs W struggled with her insomnia for a further 13 months. She said she went to bed at 11 p.m. sharp every night and turned the lights out at around 11.15 when her husband fell asleep. She would lie there in the dark with her eyes closed trying to sleep until the alarm went off at 7 a.m. She didn't feel that she slept at all during this time. She would only occasionally get out of bed to go to the toilet or to attend to her child, who by now was usually sleeping through. She went back to the GP to ask for another referral to a sleep clinic and saw a locum who had not met her before. When she explained that she had not slept at all for at least a year and a half he told her she must have been sleeping or she would have been dead.

2. Was the GP correct?

Yes, although humans can go for several days at a time without sleep, total sleep deprivation in animal experiments was rapidly fatal.

Mrs W was incensed by the doctor's response, became verbally aggressive and threw a box of tissues against the wall before storming out of the surgery. The GP referred her to the community mental health team for a psychiatric review, but they confirmed that, aside from the insomnia, there was no sign of any psychiatric disorder. They referred her to the insomnia clinic and discharged her.

When we saw her in the insomnia clinic we were faced with a difficult dilemma. The GP was correct in saying she must have been getting some sleep. However, Mrs W was clearly not going to believe that and if we told her the same, we might risk permanently damaging the therapeutic relationship. We therefore explained to her that she was clearly not getting enough sleep, as evidenced by the fact that she was feeling tired and irritable during the day. We explained that some people do have very brief, broken episodes of sleep which they will not necessarily be subjectively aware of. We then broached the possibility that this may be the case for her, but that whether it was or not, we still felt she had an insomnia that needed treating. She was adamant that we were wrong, but was willing to engage with us, as we promised to fully investigate and treat her insomnia.

We asked her first of all to keep a sleep diary to record her times in bed. She recorded a very regular bedtime of 11 p.m., but as the diary was done during the school holidays, her rising time was very variable, ranging from 7 a.m. to 11 a.m. She reported no sleep during the two weeks that she kept the diary. She insisted she needed a brain scan, but we explained that this was unlikely to tell us anything useful. We did, however, refer her for an overnight polysomnogram. This showed a total sleep time of 6 hours 22 minutes! She fell asleep after 46 minutes, spent little time in deep slow wave sleep and had 16 awakenings during the night. Her wakefulness after sleep onset was 52 minutes.

3. What is her diagnosis?

Mrs W clearly has sleep initiation and sleep maintenance insomnia, and this explains her daytime tiredness. But what is most striking is that despite this, she is actually getting a significant amount of sleep. She therefore has paradoxical insomnia or sleep state misperception—she is asleep without being aware that she is asleep. This is not at all uncommon in insomnia patients, who frequently significantly underestimate their TST. This is probably because patients with insomnia self-monitor a great deal. They are constantly monitoring whether they are awake or asleep, whether they are feeling sleepy, etc. As a result, they will be more aware of their awakenings, noises and other external stimuli, and will remember them the next morning. Good sleepers may also wake several times a night, hear noises, etc., but as they are not self-monitoring they do not remember it the next day. The insomniac presumes that because they were aware of these things they must have been awake and will mentally string the moments of awareness together, thus perceiving themselves to have been awake for extended periods.

Indeed, there are cases of pure paradoxical insomnia where people will objectively sleep very well but believe they have not slept at all. They may not have daytime symptoms, but are extremely distressed by their perceived lack of sleep. This sleep state misperception can sometimes be extremely resistant to treatment and patients can remain convinced of their sleeplessness even in the face of clear objective evidence to the contrary. However, as many patients can have genuine insomnia and sleep state misperception, one should not dismiss patients who report that they do not sleep at all without fully investigating them.

Mrs W received a copy of her polysomnogram report in the mail prior to her follow-up appointment and called the clinic to say she was insulted by the report and demanded an explanation. We showed her the full polysomnogram report, and explained in detail how the polysomnogram was scored and that there was no doubt that she had slept for a significant period of time. We explained the diagnosis of paradoxical insomnia and how we think it develops. Once again, we stressed that she did also have genuine insomnia, that we took her concerns seriously and that we intended to treat her.

4. How would you treat paradoxical insomnia?

This is an area that has not been particularly well researched. As a rule, the treatment tends to be the same as for any other insomnia complaint, i.e. hypnotics and/or CBT for insomnia. Showing the patient their polysomnogram results can be therapeutic for many patients and is sufficient to reassure them that they are sleeping. If this is not sufficient, it can sometimes be very helpful to show the patient the raw tracing of their polysomnogram and for the technician to score the polysomnogram with the patient. This obviously involves showing them how to differentiate between the waking EEG and the sleep EEG. There has been a small case series showing success with this approach. It can also be helpful if the PSG is accompanied by a video, as some paradoxical insomnia patients are convinced that the tracing must belong to another patient! We were unable to do this with Mrs W, as the polysomnogram was done in a different hospital.

We therefore needed to find another way of convincing her she was sleeping. We asked her to get a golf score counter. This records the number of times a button is pressed. We asked her to do something we would normally discourage, which is to watch the clock. We asked her to press the counter every half an hour on the half hour. As she was in bed for eight hours, if she was awake for all this time we would expect the counter to record 16 presses. She did this for a week and found that the number of clicks ranged from four to nine. She therefore became aware that she had 'lost time' 'at various points during the night. She conceded that she may therefore have fallen asleep for a few minutes at a time'. We also asked her to do something else that we normally discourage, which was to listen to an audiobook in bed. She admitted that although she felt she had not slept, she had 'lost' a few chapters here and there during the night and therefore probably had nodded off.

As Mrs W had already tried hypnotics without any success, we decided to concentrate our efforts on using cognitive behavioural techniques. She joined a CBT for insomnia group and engaged well with this. One of the core techniques of CBT for insomnia is sleep scheduling, which involves very closely matching the time in bed to the actual time asleep (see case study 48). Patients keep a sleep diary for a week and work out their average sleep time. They then ensure they do not spend any longer in bed than their average sleep time. As Mrs W recorded her sleep time as 0 minutes every night, it was very useful having the polysomnogram, and so we set her maximum time in bed as 6 hours 25 minutes. This meant she was going to bed no earlier than 00.35. As she was staying up later, she started to experience subjective sleepiness when she was trying to stay awake until her new bedtime. This made her feel more confident that she was actually likely to get some sleep. We also instructed her in the technique of Paradoxical Intent. This involves doing everything exactly as one would on any other night, keeping to the normal bedtime routine, going to bed and then trying to stay awake with the eyes open. This can be a very effective technique, probably because it stops the person from striving for sleep. This removes much of the anxiety they experience and can lead to more rapid sleep onset. But in Mrs W's case it had the added benefit that she really struggled to keep her eyes open for more than a few minutes and this allowed to her to subjectively experience her increasing level of sleepiness.

After two weeks Mrs W reported that she felt she was starting to have more extended periods of sleep. She still felt that her sleep time was under 4 hours in total, but was elated that she was making progress. She also noticed that she was less irritable and tired during the day. She was never entirely convinced that she had been sleeping all along, but, as she was clearly improving, we didn't feel it necessary to pursue the point any further.

Learning points

Paradoxical insomnia or sleep state misperception is a condition where the person sleeps without subjectively feeling they have slept. A certain degree of sleep state misperception is common in insomnia.

Some patients will be very reassured when shown objective evidence that they have slept while others are very set in their beliefs.

Complete sleeplessness for more than a few days at a time is not compatible with life and so everyone gets some sleep.

It is tempting to dismiss claims of complete sleeplessness, but paradoxical insomnia can cause significant distress and should be addressed. If there are no daytime symptoms, then helping the patient to become aware of their sleep is the only treatment required. If there are daytime symptoms, then it should be treated in the same way as any other insomnia.

Further reading

Geyer JD et al. Sleep education for paradoxical insomnia. Behavioral Sleep Medicine 2011 Jan;9(4):266–72.

needed to be addressed in order for her to improve. Nevertheless, she agreed to try an antidepressant and was put on a succession of selective serotonin reuptake inhibitors and tricyclic antidepressants, without any benefit. She also tried over-the-counter antihistamines, which only worked for a few nights and made her feel drowsy during the day. Herbal remedies, lavender oil in her bath and an expensive new mattress did not improve her sleep.

In an attempt to get more sleep, she decided that she would reduce her evening work commitments further so she could go to bed earlier. She reasoned that this would give her more opportunity to sleep. She therefore started going to bed at 10.00 p.m., but found that she would often lie awake for two hours rather than one before falling asleep. If she did manage to fall asleep earlier, she found that her sleep was lighter and more fragmented than before. She felt that her sleep was therefore deteriorating and became increasingly anxious about it. This anxiety led to a further deterioration in both her sleep and her mood.

Questions

1 Why did her sleep get worse rather than better when she spent longer in bed?

2 What investigation would be most useful in this case?

3 What is her mean sleep onset latency (SOL), total sleep time (TST), wakefulness after sleep onset (WASO) and sleep efficiency (SE)? How do these compare to normal values?

4 How do we calculate the threshold time and increase SE?

5 How do we adjust the sleep schedule over time?

Answers

1. Why did her sleep get worse rather than better when she spent longer in bed?

It is a common belief amongst insomnia sufferers that they need to give themselves more opportunity to sleep and that they should therefore spend as long as possible in bed. However, this is often a counterproductive strategy. They rarely get any more sleep than they did before and therefore the extra time in bed (TIB) is largely spent awake. This strengthens the association between the bed and wakefulness, and reinforces the belief that they are a poor sleeper. This leads to increased anxiety about sleep and they find themselves in a downward spiral.

During the day we gradually build up fatigue until we reach a threshold where the fatigue is sufficient to allow us to sleep through the night. Insomnia sufferers usually go to bed long before they have reached that threshold time. Hence they have to lie in bed awake until they reach the threshold time. Sometimes they will be able to fall asleep early, but as they have not yet built up enough fatigue to sleep through the night, they tend to wake up very early.

2. What investigation would be most useful in this case?

Laboratory investigations such as polysomnograms are generally not indicated in insomnia unless there is a suspicion from the history that there is another comorbid sleep disorder. A good history is usually sufficient to make a diagnosis of insomnia as well as elucidating the underlying cause. However, a sleep diary is often very helpful. It allows you to look at more than one night and pick up patterns that are not always evident from the history. It also allows you to work out a number of important parameters such as TIB, TST, SOL, number of awakenings, WASO and SE. In patients who have excessive sleepiness, it allows you to determine whether they are giving themselves adequate sleep opportunity.

Mrs C kept a sleep diary for two weeks. The diary for the second week is shown in Table 48.1.

Table 48.1 Baseline sleep diary of a patient with insomnia

Week starting:	Last night I went to bed at:	This morning I got up at:	So I was in bed for? minutes: (TIB)	It took me? minutes to fall asleep: (SOL)	I woke? times:	During the night I was awake for? minutes: (WASO)	In total I think I slept for? minutes: (TST)	Other info.:
Night 1	10:00	7:00	540	120	3	85	335	
Night 2	10:05	9:15	670	120	3	180	370	Felt very hot
Night 3	10:00	7:00	540	100	4	130	310	
Night 4	10:00	9:00	660	130	3	170	360	Argument with Ben
Night 5	10:30	7:00	510	90	2	60	360	
Night 6	10:40	9:00	620	180	3	130	310	Drank too much!
Night 7	10:00	11:30	810	180	4	195	435	
Total			4,350	920	22	950	2,480	
Average in minutes			**B** 621	131	3.1	136	**A** 354	
Average in hours and minutes							**C** 5 hours 55 minutes (rounded to nearest 5 minutes)	

A ÷ B x 100 = SE

354 ÷ 621 x 100 = 57%

3. **What are her mean SOL, TST, WASO and SE? How do these compare to normal values?**

While there are no clear quantitative criteria for normal sleep, it is generally considered that an SOL of less than 30 minutes, a WASO of less than 30 minutes and an SE of above 85% are normal. Mrs C's SOL is 131 minutes, and so she clearly has sleep initiation insomnia. Her WASO (the amount of time she is awake during the night, not counting the time it took her to fall asleep in the first place) is elevated at 136. She therefore has sleep maintenance insomnia as well. Her TST is 5 hours 55 minutes. There is no normal value for TST. Everyone has a different sleep need and the TST that is normal for each individual is the amount of sleep that person needs to feel well and alert most of the day on most days. SE is a measure of what proportion of the time one is in bed is actually spent asleep and this expressed as a percentage. Mrs C is in bed for an average of 621 minutes, but only 354 minutes are actually spent asleep. Therefore, her SE is 354/621 x 100 = 57%. This is low and indicates that she is spending an excessive amount of TIB awake. As she is spending 43% of the TIB awake, this pattern will strengthen her association between the bed and the insomnia. It will also increase the opportunity for her to have brief, light dozes, which will reduce the homeostatic drive for sleep, thus leading to light, broken sleep. We therefore want to ensure that she goes to bed close to the threshold time when she has built up adequate fatigue and had a strong homeostatic sleep drive, and we want to increase her SE so that she spends a minimum amount of TIB awake.

4. **How do we calculate the threshold time and increase SE?**

The first step is to establish a set rising time for Mrs C. She should keep to this rising time 7 days a week, whether she has slept well or slept badly. It is far more important to keep a set rising time than a set bedtime. As Mrs C has to rise at 7.00 a.m. three days a week, we set this as her rising time. We then calculated her average TST (5 hours 55 minutes) and subtracted this from her rising time. This gave us a threshold time of 1.05 a.m. (Note: if the patient's TST is less than five hours, we set the threshold time at five hours before the rising time.)

Table 48.2 Sleep diary at the start of sleep scheduling

Week starting:	Last night I went to bed at:	This morning I got up at:	So I was in bed for? minutes: (TIB)	It took me? minutes to fall asleep: (SOL)	I woke? times:	During the night I was awake for? minutes: (WASO)	In total I think I slept for? minutes: (TST)	Other info.:
Night 1	1:10	7:00	350	15	2	15	320	
Night 2	1:05	7:00	355	10	0	0	345	Slept through!
Night 3	1:20	7:00	340	10	1	10	320	
Night 4	1:05	7:00	355	35	3	25	295	Stressed at work
Night 5	1:05	7:00	355	5	2	10	340	
Night 6	1:05	7:00	355	10	1	3	342	
Night 7	1:05	7:00	355	2	2	15	338	
Total			2,465	87	12	78	2,300	
Average in minutes			**B** 352	12	1.7	11	**A** 328	
Average in hours and minutes							**C** 5 hours 28 minutes (rounded to nearest 5 minutes)	

A ÷ B x 100 = SE

328 ÷ 352 x 100 = 93%

We then advised Mrs C that she should not go to bed until:

1. she had reached her threshold time; and
2. she was feeling sleepy.

This rapidly increased her SE. Because she was staying up much later, she was feeling very sleepy by the time she got into bed and therefore, with the exception of the first few nights when she was still feeling anxious about the reduced TIB, she fell asleep quickly. She also found that her sleep was deeper and her awakenings were fewer and briefer.

Her sleep diary on the second week after starting sleep scheduling is shown in Table 48.2. Note that, although her TST has dropped, she is falling asleep quickly and having very little wakefulness after sleep onset. Her SE is now excellent at 93%.

5. How do we adjust the sleep schedule over time?

Mrs C continued to keep a sleep diary every week and calculated her SE at the end of each week. The SE she achieved each week determined the threshold time for the following week:

- If her sleep efficiency is less than 85%, she should move her threshold time for the following week 15 minutes later (but not going below the five hours minimum).
- If her sleep efficiency is 85–89%, she should keep her threshold time the same for the following week.
- If her sleep efficiency was 90% or above, she should move her threshold time 15 minutes earlier.

By keeping a sleep diary and making the relevant adjustments every week, Mrs C gradually increased her TIB and her TST, while maintaining a good SE. Her diary at three months is shown in Table 48.3. Her TST had increased to 7 hours 10 minutes and her SE was 98%. The improvement in sleep was reflected in improved daytime symptoms. Her mood was much improved and she stopped her antidepressant.

She had the occasional bad night and the odd day when she felt tired and irritable, but was reassured that this is normal. This

Table 48.3 Sleep diary three months after sleep scheduling

Week starting:	Last night I went to bed at:	This morning I got up at:	So I was in bed for? minutes:(TIB)	It took me? minutes to fall asleep:(SOL)	I woke? times:	During the night I was awake for? minutes:(WASO)	In total I think I slept for? minutes:(TST)	Other info.:
Night 1	11:4C	7:00	440	5	1	5	430	
Night 2	11:30	7:00	450	10	1	5	435	Slept through!
Night 3	11:45	7:00	435	5	0	0	430	
Night 4	11:40	7:00	440	5	1	5	430	Stressed at work
Night 5	12:05	7:00	415	5	0	0	410	
Night 6	11:30	7:00	450	10	0	0	440	
Night 7	11:30	7:00	450	5	1	10	435	
Total			3,080	45	4	25	3,010	
Average in minutes			**B** 440	6	0.6	4	**A** 430	
Average in hours and minutes							**C** 7 hours 10 minutes (rounded to nearest 5 minutes)	

A ÷ B x 100 = SE

430 ÷ 440 x 100 = 98%

is not a minor point. When someone has been suffering from insomnia for a long time they will often come to believe that good sleepers sleep well every night and feel alert and refreshed all day every day. It is important to remind them that even the best sleepers have occasional bad nights and will have days, or periods during the day, when they feel tired. This ensures they have realistic expectations and also means they are less likely to panic if they have a bad night.

Once she had settled into her new sleep schedule she no longer felt the need to keep a diary and she felt much less anxious about her sleep. She still has a lie-in on some Sunday mornings and is aware that this may mean she will have slightly poorer sleep on Sunday night, but she is confident that her sleep will return to normal on Monday when she keeps to her 7.00 a.m. wake-up time.

Learning points

What precipitates insomnia and what perpetuates it are not necessarily the same thing. Insomnia is often triggered by a defined stressor, but it often persists once the stressor has been removed. This is largely due to anxiety and dysfunctional sleep habits.

Most insomnia sufferers spend more TIB to give themselves more opportunity to sleep. This rarely works, as it simply extends the amount of wakefulness in bed and ultimately makes the insomnia worse.

Patients should be encouraged to rise at the same time every day. Anchoring the rising time is much more important than keeping a regular bedtime. In fact, keeping a regular bedtime can be counterproductive. Patients should only go to bed when sleepy. If they keep their rising time the same, they will naturally start to feel sleepy at the same time each evening.

Using a sleep diary to calculate the patient's average TST one can work out the threshold time (in practice the *earliest* bedtime) for the patient. They should not go to bed until they have reached their threshold time and are sleepy. As their sleep improves, their threshold can be moved forward.

Further reading

Morin C, Espie C. Insomnia: a clinical guide to assessment and treatment. 2003; Springer, New York.

Perlis M et al. Cognitive behavioral treatment of insomnia: a session-by-session guide. 2005; Springer, New York.

Case 49
A sleep cycle that keeps moving

Dr L is a 32-year-old musicologist who presented to the sleep clinic with a very chaotic sleep pattern. He would have periods of a week or two of sleeping reasonably well, followed by a week or two of having significant difficulty getting to sleep until the early hours of the morning. He also reported having nights where he would not sleep at all. If he slept well, he felt alert and well during the day. When his sleep was significantly delayed, or he did not get any sleep at all, he would be very sleepy during the day and would fall asleep on the train on his way to and from work, as well as at work. Some of these daytime naps could last for several hours if he was not disturbed and this made it even harder for him to fall asleep at night.

He had been sleeping in this pattern for most of his adult life. When he was a student his timetable was flexible enough that he was able to work around it, but since starting work as a lecturer his daytime commitments became more set and he found it extremely difficult to cope. As a result he went to the GP, who prescribed hypnotics. He found these helpful when he was going through a period of poor sleep, but still felt sleepier during the day than when he was having a period of good sleep.

On taking a full sleep history Dr L commented that his sleep cycle had evolved with time. When he was writing his PhD thesis he worked from home for a period of 6 months and had very few external commitments. During this time he noticed that his overall sleep time was better. However, he found that his sleep period would become progressively later each day. As a result, he would fall asleep later and wake up later each day and his sleep would gradually rotate around the clock. When he allowed his sleep cycle to drift around the clock in this manner he was reasonably alert during his wake period and able to concentrate on his work. However, when he was going through periods of sleeping during the day and working through the night he felt socially quite isolated and his mood suffered as a result.

Questions

1 What is the likely diagnosis?

2 Which group of patients are at high risk of non-24-hour sleep–wake syndrome?

3 What investigation would you use to confirm the diagnosis?

4 How would you treat this?

history. The data is presented in both numerical and visual form, making it easy to see how the sleep–wake cycle evolves over time.

The patient's actigraph is shown in Figure 49.1. The black spikes indicate movement and therefore wakefulness, whilst the white areas with little or no movement activity represent sleep. You can see a clear trend towards progressive delay of the sleep period, thus confirming the diagnosis of a non-24-hour sleep–wake syndrome.

4. How would you treat this?

Treatment of non-24-hour sleep–wake syndrome involves using melatonin and, where possible, light to stabilize the circadian rhythm. As the trend is for the sleep–wake cycle to be progressively delayed, the melatonin and light need to be timed in such a way as to counter this delay, i.e. they should advance the cycle. If the regime is successfully implemented, the body's tendency to delay the cycle will be balanced by the treatment's tendency to advance it.

The timing of the melatonin and light is essential for successful treatment. For example, if the melatonin is given too late it will not pull the patient's cycle forward and their natural propensity to drift later will not be adequately opposed. If the melatonin is taken too early it may in fact fall at a point in their cycle where it is ineffective or even accelerates their phase delay, thus pulling their circadian rhythm in the wrong direction. The timing of melatonin is particularly crucial in blind patients, as they cannot use light and so they have only one treatment available to them.

It is also important to note that not all light is equally effective in influencing circadian rhythms—it is particularly light in the blue–green part of the spectrum. The ideal light to use is natural daylight, but obviously this is not always practical. Therefore, patients usually use a SAD lamp. These lights are designed to be particularly intense in the blue–green wavelengths. Patients do not have to stare at the light, but the light should be placed directly in front of the patient and should be reasonably close to them. They can read, watch the TV behind the light, etc. In most applications it is advised that the patient use it for 30–60 minutes depending on the intensity of the light and their individual response to it.

We allowed Dr L's cycle to rotate until he was falling asleep and waking up at the desired time. When he was falling asleep at 11.00 p.m. and waking at 7.00 a.m. he started taking melatonin in the late afternoon and used bright light for an hour immediately on waking. This held his cycle stable for long periods of time and his daytime symptoms improved significantly. Ten months after starting treatment he had a month's holiday and decided to stop the melatonin and light to see what would happen. He very rapidly returned to his non-24-hour sleep–wake cycle, but on restarting the treatment he was able to reinstate an entrained circadian rhythm. He experienced some mild headaches from time to time in the mornings, which could have been a side effect of either the melatonin or the light, but otherwise reported no side effects.

Learning points

Non-24-hour sleep–wake syndrome is characterized by a circadian rhythm that is progressively delayed, leading to the sleep period getting later and later, ultimately rotating around the clock.

It is particularly common in blind patients and should always be screened for in this population.

Treatment involves stabilizing the circadian rhythm with carefully timed melatonin and, if possible, daylight.

Where daylight is not an option, a SAD light can be used.

Circadian rhythm disorders can be masked by hypnotics, lifestyle and work pressures, and so it is important to enquire about periods of time when these were not impinging on the patient's natural sleep cycle.

Further reading

Ancoli-Israel S et al. The role of actigraphy in the study of sleep and circadian rhythms. Sleep 2003 May;26(3):342–92.

Uchiyama M, Lockley SW. Non-24-hour sleep–wake syndrome in sighted and blind patients. Sleep Med Clin 2009 Jun;4(2):195–211.

Case 50
My body is in London but my body clock is in New York

Mr V is a 21-year-old college student who presented to the clinic with a history of severe initial insomnia. Starting from around the age of 15 years he has had increasing difficulty getting to sleep at night. He would go to bed at around 11 p.m. every night, but found it impossible to get to sleep before 3.00 or 4.00 a.m. During term time he would rise with great difficulty to three alarms and much prompting from his increasingly frustrated parents in order to get to class on time. He struggled with concentration during class, frequently falling asleep, particularly in morning lessons. His concentration and alertness improved in the afternoon, though he was still very tired. Despite his fatigue he found himself becoming progressively more alert in the evening and felt most awake around 12.00–1.00 a.m. He became progressively more depressed and was seen by several child and adolescent psychiatrists. He had some psychotherapy, which improved his relationship with his parents but did not improve his mood or his sleep pattern.

On completing school he took a gap year and worked as a DJ in a nightclub, working from around 10 p.m. to 3 a.m. He then slept from 4 a.m. through to midday and felt much more alert when awake. He also noticed a significant improvement in his mood. However, since starting college he has had to start waking at 8.00 a.m., but has not been able to move his time of sleep onset any earlier than 3.00 a.m. He therefore only sleeps five hours a night at most and has started to struggle at college. His depression has also returned.

Questions

1 What is the likely diagnosis?

2 Why did he feel tired in the morning despite sleeping better on the hypnotic?

3 What investigations would you do to confirm the diagnosis?

4 How do you treat delayed sleep phase syndrome (DSPS)?

5 Are there any other treatments for DSPS?

Answers

1. What is the likely diagnosis?

This history is typical of a DSPS. This is a circadian rhythm disorder where the person has a normal 24-hour sleep–wake cycle, but their internal biological clock is delayed relative to the outside world— 'their body is in London but their body clock is in New York'. They have the same fluctuations in alertness that normal people have, but they occur later. Therefore, they are still feeling very alert late at night when the rest of the world is going to bed, and they only start to feel the normal late-night sleepiness in the early hours of the morning. They have difficulty staying awake in the mornings, as this is their time of lowest alertness—10 or 11 a.m. for someone with DSPS is the equivalent of 4–5 a.m. for everyone else. Similarly, the late evening for someone with DSPS is the equivalent of the after-noon for everyone else, and so it is no surprise that it is difficult for them to initiate sleep at this time. DSPS is more common in adoles-cents and young adults, though it can occur in any age group. The fact that it is much more common in adolescents than in adults in-dicates that most people will grow out of DSPS. Around one in ten patients presenting with insomnia may in fact have DSPS and it is important to exclude this disorder in any patient who presents with sleep onset insomnia.

Mr V tried numerous remedies over the years, with very little suc-cess. He tried going to bed earlier, but found he simply lay awake until 3–4 a.m. regardless of what time he went to bed. He tried stay-ing up for 36 hours to reset his cycle, and while he sometimes man-aged to fall asleep in the evening on the first night after doing this, by the second night he had reverted to his usual pattern. In desper-ation he asked the GP for hypnotics. He was given a prescription, but was advised only to use them if absolutely necessary. He found he was able to get to sleep at a normal time with the hypnotic and sleep through the night, but still felt very sleepy in the morning. As soon as he stopped the medication, he reverted to his delayed sleep pattern.

2. Why did he feel tired in the morning despite sleeping better on the hypnotic?

The tiredness that patients with DSPS feel in the morning has two causes. The first is that, as they cannot fall asleep until late, they are sleep deprived. The other reason is that their circadian alertness drive is at its minimum in the morning and the timing of the circadian clock is not directly affected by sleep. So even if they get an adequate quantity of sleep on a hypnotic, their body clock will still be delayed. Therefore, they will feel the same in the mid-morning period as others would at around 5 a.m. regardless of how much they have slept. However, as the day progresses and their circadian alertness drive increases, their alertness will improve. Indeed, this is what Mr V reported. The hypnotic did not make him feel any better in the morning, but he did feel better later in the day, as he was not sleep deprived.

3. What investigations would you do to confirm the diagnosis?

The diagnosis of DSPS is largely made on history. However, it can be useful to get the patient to fill in a sleep diary and to perform a few weeks of wrist actigraphy. The actigraph measures movement and can give an objective longitudinal view of the patient's sleep pattern in the real world. If possible, it is helpful to do the actigraphy during a period where they allow themselves to sleep in their natural rhythm, as well as during a period when the patient is working, going to college, etc. and is therefore having to get up in the morning. By monitoring the sleep pattern when they are sleeping in their natural rhythm one can see what that rhythm is, and it also allows one to exclude initial insomnia. If the patient has initial insomnia rather than a DSPS, one would expect to see delayed sleep onset on the actigraph but not necessarily a delay in the rising time. Doing some of the actigraphy when the patient is trying to get up in the morning gives one an idea of how much less sleep they get in these circumstances, which can be useful when advocating on their behalf with work, school, etc.

4. How do you treat DSPS?

As the underlying cause of DSPS is a delay in the internal circadian clock relative to the outside world, the main aim of treatment is to advance that circadian clock. Although there is some complex neural circuitry driving the clock, the clock can be mediated using melatonin and light. Melatonin 'pulls' the sleep cycle towards itself while light 'pushes' it away. Thus in order to advance the clock one needs to take melatonin before sleep to pull the sleep forward and use light after sleep to push the sleep period earlier.

The timing of the melatonin and light is critical. The times of maximum effect are calculated relative to the person's natural dim light melatonin onset (DLMO). The DLMO is the time that the person starts secreting melatonin when in a dark environment. However, the DLMO is very rarely used in clinical settings—because the time of the DLMO will move as the therapy starts to take effect, one would need to do it repeatedly and this is not practical. (For more information on how the DLMO is determined, see Case Study 46 (ASPS)). Therefore, we need to estimate the time of the DLMO from the person's sleep onset time. A good rule of thumb is that the DLMO tends to occur two hours before sleep onset and the best time to give melatonin is about six hours before sleep onset. Obviously one cannot predict the time of sleep onset, so we use the time of sleep onset the night before. Thus the person takes melatonin approximately six hours earlier than the time of sleep onset (NB: time of sleep onset, not the time they went to bed) the night before. They then get exposure to light, either by going outdoors or using a seasonal affective disorder (SAD) lamp immediately on waking for 30–60 minutes. (See Case Study 49 for more detail on how to use light.) This will gradually pull the sleep cycle forward.

Mr V instituted this regime and found that his sleep cycle gradually advanced over a period of two weeks until it eventually settled into a pattern where he was falling asleep at midnight and waking at 8.00 a.m. He was therefore taking his melatonin at 6.00 p.m. Even more striking was that his depression rapidly resolved and his performance at college improved, as he was much more alert during the morning classes.

5. Are there any other treatments for DSPS?

Chronotherapy is an alternative technique that is sometimes used. Trying to go to bed earlier each night is a strategy that rarely, if ever, works. But doing the opposite can be quite effective. The patient sets aside a week or two to undergo the chronotherapy and they then go to bed an hour or two later each day. This means their period of wakefulness is longer than usual and so it is much easier to initiate sleep. As a result, their sleep–wake cycle becomes progressively delayed until they are sleeping in phase with the outside world. Once this happens, the chronotherapy is stopped and the regime with melatonin and light is instituted to hold the person in phase.

Learning points

DSPS is a common condition, particularly in adolescents and young adults. It is an important differential diagnosis for initial insomnia.

The mainstay of treatment is to advance the circadian rhythm using evening melatonin and morning light. The timing of both melatonin and light is critical.

An alternative treatment is chronotherapy, which involves progressively delaying sleep until the person is falling asleep and waking up at the desired time; however, once they are sleeping in phase, they may need melatonin and light to hold them in phase.

Some patients may choose professions that allow them to start work late and finish late, thus altering their lifestyle to fit their circadian rhythm. However, they should be aware that they may grow out of the DSPS with time.

Further reading

Morgenthaler TI et al. Practice parameters for the clinical evaluation and treatment of circadian rhythm sleep disorders. An American Academy of Sleep Medicine report. Sleep 2007 Dec;30(11):1445–59.

Van Geijlswijk IM, Korzilius HPLM, Smits MG. The use of exogenous melatonin in delayed sleep phase disorder: a meta-analysis. Sleep 2010 Dec;33(12):1605–14.

5. Are there any other treatments for DSPS?

Chronotherapy is an alternative to light therapy which is sometimes used. Trying to go to bed earlier each night is a strategy that rarely, if ever, works. But doing the opposite can be quite effective. The patient sets aside a week or two to undergo the chronotherapy and they then go to bed an hour or two later each night until their period of wakefulness is longer than usual... it is far easier to initiate...

Case 51
A very, very long day

Mr L is a 63-year-old engineer who presented to the sleep clinic with a life-long complaint of very short sleep. He remembers as a child that his parents would put him to bed at 8 p.m. every night and he would lie awake for hours before falling asleep. He would then wake very early in the morning and when he was going to school, he would be up, dressed and finished breakfast before his father, a bus conductor, left for work at 6 a.m.

Initially he tried to increase his sleep time by staying in bed with the lights off, but he found this increasingly frustrating and took to reading with a pocket torch until his parents fell asleep, at which point he would turn the light on and read until he felt sleepy. He felt this sleep pattern actually gave him an advantage over his classmates, as he was able to read and study for several hours more each day. His parents, however, were extremely concerned about how the lack of sleep would affect him and they took him to a succession of doctors, some of whom prescribed antihistamines as hypnotics. These did increase his sleep time, but he always felt groggy the next day and his sleep returned to baseline as soon as the course of medication was finished.

When Mr L went to university he had to work a late-night job to fund his studies while attending classes during the day. He found this fairly easy, as he only slept five hours a night and felt alert and focused during the day. He did not feel particularly anxious about his short sleep, as many of his peers were burning the candle at both ends, though they generally needed to nap during the day to maintain that lifestyle. Indeed his sleep was not an issue until he got married in his thirties. His wife would sleep eight hours a night, and he naturally tried to go to bed at the same time and rise at the same time as her. However, he was never able to match her sleep time and he and his wife became increasingly anxious about his relative lack of sleep. Once again he was tried on a number of hypnotics and sedative antidepressants. These increased his sleep time slightly, but the daytime fatigue he experienced led him to discontinue all of them.

As he grew older his sleep time gradually reduced from five hours to three hours. He denied any daytime fatigue and indeed ran a very successful business, played tennis twice a week and was in good health. His primary complaint with his sleep pattern was that he would go to bed at the same time as his wife and lay awake feeling frustrated for most of the night. He also frequently travelled for business and would be awake for much of the night in his hotel room, feeling extremely bored. He was therefore keen to increase his sleep time to fit better with his lifestyle.

Questions

1 Does Mr L have insomnia?
2 Is it possible to be a short sleeper and have insomnia?
3 What are the causes of short sleep?
4 How would you treat Mr L?

in the initial assessment, he was afraid that his short sleep was some-how damaging him, or a sign that he was abnormal.

However, he still wished he could sleep longer. We agreed to give him a course of cognitive behaviour therapy for insomnia (CBT-I), which he found useful although it didn't increase his sleep time. As part of the CBT-I we taught him sleep scheduling and explained that he should not go to bed earlier than five hours before his rising time. He should also not go to bed until he was feeling sleepy. His wife was very anxious about this routine, and so we invited her to attend the clinic with Mr L so we could explain the rationale behind this ap-proach and help them work out, as a couple, how to accommodate this new schedule without disrupting their relationship or Mrs L's sleep. They reached a compromise whereby Mr L would go to bed with his wife and stay with her until she fell asleep. He would then get up and use the extra time in his day to engage in relaxing, enjoyable activities and going back to bed when he reached his threshold time and was sleepy.

At follow-up Mr L was feeling much less anxious about his sleep. He said it was a relief not to feel that he had to spend eight hours in bed and remarked that at age 63 he had at last been given permission to stay up late. His only complaint was that now he had so much more time in the day that he was struggling to find things to occupy him for his 21 hours of wakefulness. However, on balance he felt it was not a bad problem to have. Although his total sleep time had not increased at all, as he was no longer distressed about his sleep he no longer had insomnia.

Learning points

There is no 'right' amount of sleep. Each person's needs are different (and can change with time). The common perception that we all need eight hours' sleep is not true. The acid test is how the person feels dur-ing the day. If they are alert and feel well most of the day most days, they are getting enough sleep for them.

However, one can be a short sleeper and have insomnia on top of the short sleep. Indeed the constant striving by short sleepers to achieve the mythical ideal of eight hours' sleep may raise their anxiety and precipitate the insomnia.

There are three reasons why someone may be a short sleeper. Some people simply need less sleep (short sleepers), some need more sleep but are prevented from getting it by lifestyle or environmental factors (sleep deprivation), and some need more sleep but are unable to get it despite adequate opportunity and the absence of environmental factors (insomnia).

If someone is a short sleeper but does not have daytime symptoms, then reassurance that they are getting as much as sleep as they need is often the only intervention they require.

Further reading

Chesson A et al. Practice parameters for the evaluation of chronic insomnia: an American Academy of Sleep Medicine report. Sleep 2000;23:237–41.

Case 52
Sleep and alcohol abuse

Mr O is a 39-year-old unemployed ex-soldier who was referred to the Insomnia Clinic from the local alcohol treatment team. He had been drinking heavily for 11 years and had undergone two previous in-patient detoxes followed by residential rehabilitation programmes. However, he was unable to remain abstinent for more than a few weeks after each detox. He initially returned to drinking at night, but this rapidly escalated to daytime and then morning drinking as well. He was scheduled to have a third attempt at detoxification and rehabilitation. He felt that this was his last chance and was very motivated to make a success of it. His key worker spent considerable time with him discussing why the previous attempts had failed and what could be done to increase his chances of success this time around. He explained that when he was discharged from the army he struggled to settle back into civilian life and was unable to find a job. He became increasingly anxious and frustrated, and therefore developed sleep initiation insomnia. He sought help from his GP, who gave him sleep hygiene advice. When this did not help, his GP prescribed a short course of hypnotics, which he found very effective. However, when he went back to the GP to ask for more, his GP refused, expressing concerns that he might become addicted to them. Mr O became increasingly fatigued from his insomnia, which made it harder to look for work or engage socially with others. He started drinking in the evenings to initiate sleep. He found that this helped him to get off to sleep, though he still felt tired during the day. Over the next two years he gradually had to increase the amount of alcohol he consumed in order to get to sleep, until he was drinking 6 strong lagers every night. He then found that he would wake in the middle of the night feeling anxious and be unable to get back to sleep. He started keeping a can of lager by his bed and would drink this when he woke during the night so he could get back to sleep. He also found that he was able to sleep better during the day and so started going to bed around 6 a.m., rising at around 6 p.m., though he felt he was only asleep for six of the twelve hours in bed. His drinking continued to escalate until he was drinking almost constantly when awake.

When he had his detoxifications he was able to come off the alcohol with the cover of chlordiazepoxide and zopiclone. However, when he moved to the rehabilitation unit the medications where stopped. He very rapidly found that his sleep deteriorated. He had great difficulty initiating sleep, and when he did fall asleep his sleep was broken and he rarely slept more than four to five hours a night. While in the rehab unit he felt that he could cope with this, partly due to the lack of external pressures and partly due to the company of the other patients who were experiencing similar problems. However, when he left the rehab unit he found his sleep increasingly problematic. He found being awake for long periods at night in his hostel room frustrating and boring, and he became anxious that his lack of sleep would make it hard for him to find work. He therefore went back to drinking, which improved his sleep in the short term. Unfortunately, he rapidly needed to escalate the dose to get the same effect and returned to his pre-treatment level of drinking within a few months.

He and his key worker therefore concluded that managing his insomnia was a vital element in the treatment of his alcohol dependence, and that if he did not address the insomnia, his chances of remaining abstinent were significantly lower.

Questions

1 What effect does alcohol have on sleep?

2 How would you treat Mr O?

3 How can one institute stimulus control when the patient lives in a single room?

Answers

1. What effect does alcohol have on sleep?

The effects of alcohol on sleep are quite complex and depend on the quantity of alcohol and the time that the alcohol is consumed. Alcohol is generally sedative and so can help with sleep onset. However, as it is metabolized quickly, the sedative effect is likely to wear off during the night. In fact, the rebound alertness experienced when alcohol leaves the system can lead to an earlier awakening than would otherwise have occurred. Therefore, alcohol can lead to less total sleep despite its sedative effects, particularly at higher doses. Furthermore, alcohol impacts on the architecture of sleep both when there is alcohol in the bloodstream and in the immediate post-elimination period. It can also worsen some sleep disorders, most notably obstructive sleep apnoea, periodic limb movements and parasomnias.

In alcohol dependence the picture is more complex still. Even when alcohol does improve sleep, many people develop tolerance to the sleep-promoting effects very rapidly. However, despite this, the rebound awakening in the second half of the night does not appear to be subject to tolerance effects. In other words, when a particular dose of alcohol is no longer sufficient to induce sleep, it will still lead to early waking. Therefore, the person will find that they need higher and higher doses of alcohol to induce sleep, yet their sleep will be disrupted, leading to the temptation to 'top up' with a drink in the middle of the night. Sleep in alcoholics is often chaotic and may occur in brief episodes scattered across the 24 hours. Sleep latency is typically delayed. In the early stage of abstinence, sleep is commonly very disrupted with reduced total sleep time, reduced slow wave sleep and disrupted REM sleep. Unfortunately, the insomnia can become a chronic problem and is a strong predictor of relapse in the long term.

2. How would you treat Mr O?

Substance misuse presents a number of challenges to effective insomnia treatment. As these patients have already demonstrated a propensity to develop addiction to a substance, there is usually a reluctance to prescribe hypnotics. In Mr O's case he has developed an addiction to a substance which acts on the benzodiazepine receptor, the same receptor at which most hypnotics act. There are certainly some alcohol misusers who do well with benzodiazepine receptor agonists, and addiction to zopiclone, for example, is less likely to cause liver or cerebellar damage than addiction to alcohol. However, it is probably wisest to avoid benzodiazepine receptor agonists as a first-line treatment.

On the other hand, it is quite common to use sedative antidepressants in this population and there is some research evidence to support this practice. As many of these patients have comorbid depression and anxiety, they are highly likely to need an antidepressant and it makes sense to use one that may help their sleep.

The second obstacle to be overcome is that many substance misusers have chaotic lifestyles with very little structure. As the behavioural treatment of insomnia relies very heavily on keeping constant rising times, avoiding napping during the day and structuring the day to maximize the chances of sleeping well, this is problematic. It is not clear to what extent the lack of structure causes the sleep problem, and thus the substance misuse, or the substance causes the lack of structure. Either way, it is vital that some structure is re-established if the patient is to recover.

A final challenge in Mr O's case which is common in, but not exclusive to, substance misusers is his accommodation. One of the vital techniques in the psychological treatment of insomnia is stimulus control. This is based on the principle of classical conditioning. If someone spends a lot of time in their bed and their bedroom awake, they come to associate the bed and bedroom with wakefulness. If this association is reinforced enough, the bed and bedroom become stimuli that elicit wakefulness. An extremely common complaint in insomnia is that the person will be sitting in front of the TV and will feel very sleepy. They then go up to bed and as they walk into the bedroom it is as if 'someone has flipped a switch' in their brain and they feel wide awake. This demonstrates how powerful this associative mechanism is. In order to counter this, stimulus control advises that the bed and bedroom should be used for sleep and sex only. All waking activities such as reading, working, talking on the phone, watching TV or exercising should be done outside the bedroom. Furthermore, if the person is not asleep within 15 minutes of going to bed they should get out of bed, get out of the bedroom and do something relaxing and pleasant. They should only go back to bed when they feel sleepy and, if they are not asleep within 15 minutes of returning to bed, they should repeat the process. Mr O lived in a hostel where he only had a single bedroom with a bed and no chair. He spent most of his waking time in his room and there was nowhere to go at night if he was observing the 15-minute rule. It was therefore challenging to find ways of instituting stimulus control techniques.

3. How can one institute stimulus control when the patient lives in a single room?

The ideal scenario is to use the bed and the bedroom for sleep and sex only. Where this is not possible there is still merit in creating a separation between the sleep space and the waking space. If the patient cannot stay out of the room during the day, they should at least endeavour to stay off the bed. We therefore encourage them to sit in a chair when they are in their room during the day and not to use the bed for eating, reading, watching TV, etc. If at all possible the patient should try to create some physical separation between the bed and the rest of the room using a screen or a curtain. In some cases this is not possible and there may be no alternative but to use the bed during the day. We then suggest using various cues to differentiate between the 'daytime' bed and the 'sleeping' bed. For example, the patient should take their pillows and duvet off the bed during the day and replace them with couch cushions, a throw, etc. during the day. At night, the cushions and throw are removed and the sleeping props put on the bed. Some patients even use a teddy bear which is placed under the bed during the day and only brought out when they are ready to go to sleep!

The first step in treating Mr O's insomnia was to set realistic expectations. We explained that insomnia can take many months to improve, particularly in the context of alcohol, and that he would need to be patient. However, we also stressed that with the right interventions there was a good chance of recovery. We gave him some individual sessions of cognitive behaviour therapy for insomnia (CBT-I) (as he was drinking during the day we felt it was not appropriate for him to join group sessions) and his key worker attended the sessions with him so she could support him and reinforce the techniques. The techniques included stimulus control, sleep scheduling, relaxation, cognitive strategies for managing anxiety and psycho-education. Initially he had difficulty putting the techniques into practice, but was able to start doing some basic stimulus control with the encouragement of his key worker (who found a plastic garden chair and folding table for him to use in his room during the day).

Mr O had an in-patient detox and was given zopiclone during the detoxification process, though this was stopped when he moved to rehabilitation. Once in rehabilitation his key worker helped him institute the CBT techniques with the cooperation of the rehab house staff. His insomnia was initially very problematic, but he noticed that it did improve gradually during the three months in rehabilitation. Unfortunately, on leaving rehab he returned to his old hostel. As it was a wet hostel he spent even more time in his room, as he was trying to avoid contact with other residents who were still drinking. His sleep started to deteriorate again and this made him anxious and low in mood. It was decided that he would benefit from an antidepressant and so he was started on trazadone, which lifted his mood and anxiety, and improved his sleep to a large extent.

After six months of abstinence, Mr O was rehoused. He felt he needed a clean break from his past and accepted the offer of a flat in a different town. It was a one-bedroom flat, but as it had a separate lounge and bedroom he found it easier to institute the stimulus control techniques. His sleep remained fragile and would deteriorate when he was under stress, but he felt more able to cope with these bad periods and felt that the trazadone provided a safety net he could turn to if he was at risk of relapse. His care was transferred to a local alcohol service and his key worker included detailed instructions on his insomnia treatment in her transfer summary so they could continue to support him if needed.

Learning points

Insomnia is a significant driver of alcohol abuse.

Although patients use alcohol to self-medicate for their insomnia, the alcohol actually makes the insomnia worse.

Insomnia can remain problematic long after abstinence is achieved and is a major risk factor for relapse.

Caution is advised when considering prescribing hypnotics to patients with substance misuse. They are not absolutely contraindicated, and there may be times when long-term hypnotic use is a safer alternative to long-term alcohol or illicit drug use. However, it is usually advisable to use medications with a lower abuse potential such as sedative antidepressants and it is always advisable to use non-medical interventions such as CBT-I.

Further reading

Arnedt JT, Conroy DA, Brower KJ. Treatment options for sleep disturbances during alcohol recovery. J Addict Dis 2007;26(4):41–54.

Kolla BP, Mansukhani MP, Schneekloth T. Pharmacological treatment of insomnia in alcohol recovery: a systematic review. Alcohol and Alcoholism 2011 Sep;46(5): 578–85.

Case 53
Choosing and using hypnotics

Mrs P was a 44-year-old married mother of two teenage boys. She worked as a head teacher and her job frequently involved both early mornings and late nights. She had been a poor sleeper for as long as she could remember, but her sleep had been particularly bad for a period of three years. She went to bed feeling exhausted, but would take one to two hours to fall asleep. Once asleep she would sleep through on some nights, but on other nights would wake up after about an hour and a half and would take 30 to 90 minutes to get back to sleep. This gave her a total sleep time of four to six hours, leaving her severely fatigued, tearful and irritable during the day.

She had used basic sleep hygiene techniques and a number of alternative remedies such as valerian, hops, lavender, hypnosis CDs, hypnotherapy, homoeopathy and acupuncture. She had spent a small fortune on an expensive mattress and pillows, high-quality sheets, blackout blinds and a white noise machine. Some of these remedies would work for a few nights, which would raise her hopes, but this made it all the more devastating when they lost their effectiveness.

With her tearfulness and irritability the GP felt that she may have depression, though Mrs P disputed this. She felt her low mood was entirely secondary to the poor sleep. On the rare nights when she did sleep well her mood was noticeably better the day after. Nevertheless, she agreed to a trial of antidepressants and the GP gave her citalopram. She persisted with this for three months, but found that, if anything, it made her sleep even worse and had no impact on her mood. The GP then switched her to clomipramine, which is a sedative antidepressant. This did improve her sleep to a small extent, but she suffered significant drowsiness during the day and so asked to be taken off the medication.

Questions

1 Are antidepressants a good choice in insomnia?

2 Should polysomnograms be a routine part of insomnia investigations?

3 How do you decide which hypnotic to use?

4 What is the point of doing CBT-I if the person is taking a hypnotic?

Table 53.1 Commonly used hypnotics and their half-lives. The wide variation in the half-lives of some substances means that it can be difficult to predict how that drug will affect an individual patient, but overall the half-lives give a reasonable idea of the relative duration of action of the various drugs and their propensity to lead to daytime sedation the next day. Clonazepam is included, as it is widely used in sleep medicine for a number of conditions including parasomnias, restless legs and sleep fragmentation.

Drug	Half-Life (hours)
Zopiclone	3.5–6.5
Zolpidem	1.5–2.5
Zaleplon	1
Temazepam	8–20
Clonazepam	30–40
Promethazine	5–14
Melatonin Modified Release	3.5–4

efficacy later in the night they are not good at maintaining sleep. However, they are less likely to cause sedation the morning after taking a dose. Longer-acting drugs are good at initiating and maintaining sleep, but are more likely to cause sedation the next day. This is particularly relevant if the person has to be alert in the morning, for example if they drive to work. Table 53.1 shows some commonly used hypnotics with their half-lives. Remember that these are the half-lives, not their duration of action. The duration of action will vary from person to person. The benefit of looking at half-lives is that they give you some indication of the relative duration when comparing the different drugs. Comparing the three 'z' drugs is a case in point. Zopiclone is the longest acting of the three and is therefore useful for sleep initiation and sleep maintenance insomnia. However, many patients complain of daytime sedation with it. It is therefore no surprise that it has been shown to have an adverse effect on driving performance the morning after taking a dose. Zolpidem has a medium duration of action and so is good for sleep onset and confers some benefit for sleep maintenance, though not to the same extent as zopiclone. However, the shorter half-life makes it safer for driving the next morning. Zaleplon is rarely used, but its extremely short duration of action makes it ideal for patients who have no difficulty getting to sleep but who wake up in the middle of the night. Zaleplon can be taken in the middle of the night and will re-establish sleep quickly, but will leave the body quickly enough that there will be little or no hangover on waking in the morning.

Additional factors to consider when choosing a hypnotic are the other side effects of each drug. For example, benzodiazepines may be more likely to exacerbate obstructive sleep apnoea, while zopiclone causes an unpleasant metallic after-taste in some (though not all) patients. Whether the risks of addiction are greater with some hypnotics than others is controversial. The addictive potential of the benzodiazepines is well established; some research suggests that the 'z' drugs may be less addictive, but not everyone is convinced of this.

We discussed the options with Mrs P and, given that she drove to work every morning, we were concerned about her using zopiclone. We decided to switch her to zolpidem 10 mg, which we felt would be sufficient to control her symptoms, as her insomnia was primarily sleep initiation insomnia and when she did wake at night it tended to be in the first half of the night. Mrs P found the zolpidem to be largely effective and she felt much more alert during the day. She was also appreciative of the fact that zolpidem does not cause the metallic after-taste. She did find that once or twice a week she would wake up earlier than usual, but was not too bothered by it.

When the summer holidays came around Mrs P asked to remain on the hypnotics. She said she felt so well on the medication that she was reluctant to stop it. She was aware of the risk of addiction, but felt that it was a risk worth taking. We agreed to continue prescribing it, with a number of conditions. First, we asked that the GP prescribe the medication so that he could monitor her use on a regular basis. We arranged to see her three monthly to review whether she still needed the medication and whether there were any adverse side effects. We advised her to try to take regular drug holidays in order to reduce the likelihood of developing tolerance to the drug. Finally, we asked her to attend a course of CBT-I.

4. What is the point of doing CBT-I if the person is taking a hypnotic?

First, it is important to remember that a hypnotic is not an anaesthetic. It is unlikely to put a patient to sleep if their physiological and psychological state is not conducive to sleep. A hypnotic should be seen as something that helps someone sleep rather than something that makes them sleep. It is not uncommon for patients to initially have a good response to a hypnotic but to then find that it becomes progressively less effective. This may be a sign of tolerance, but is often actually due to poor sleep habits. Patients may become lazy about their sleep-related behaviours, for example being erratic about their sleep schedules, having caffeine in the evening or watching TV in bed. Therefore, their behaviours counteract the effect of the medication. Doing CBT-I helps patients to optimize their sleep-related behaviours so the medication has the best chance of working.

Second, most patients prefer to sleep without medication and they are often under pressure from their GPs to discontinue their hypnotics. It is therefore important to provide them with an alternative treatment.

Mrs P found the CBT course extremely helpful. She found that when the medication was combined with the CBT she was able to sleep well on only 5 mg of zolpidem on most nights. She had not been successful in stopping the medication, but was happy with her sleep and how she felt during the day. We followed her up three monthly for a year and over that time there was no loss of efficacy or dose escalation.

Learning points

The polysomnogram is rarely useful in insomnia, unless the history suggests the presence of another sleep disorder.

Insomnia can precede and cause depression, and does not necessarily remit when the depression improves.

The most important consideration when choosing a hypnotic is the duration of action. Long half-life drugs are good for improving sleep initiation and maintenance, but can lead to daytime sedation. Shorter half-life drugs are good for sleep initiation but less so for sleep maintenance. However, they are less likely to cause daytime sedation. Always consider how important it is for the person to be alert in the morning, particularly if they drive.

When starting hypnotics it is tempting to presume that the condition is treated and nothing else needs to be done. In fact, starting a hypnotic should prompt one to redouble one's efforts to institute non-medical interventions such as CBT-I.

Further reading

Hall-Porter JM, Curry DT, Walsh JK. Pharmacologic Treatment of Primary Insomnia. Sleep Medicine Clinics 2012;5(4):609–25.

Wilson SJ et al. British Association for Psychopharmacology consensus statement on evidence-based treatment of insomnia, parasomnias and circadian rhythm disorders. Journal of Psychopharmacology 2010 Nov;24(11):1577–601.

Case 54
Please see this patient who is addicted to sleeping pills

Mr S is an accountant who presented to the clinic with a complaint of 'hypnotic addiction'. He had both sleep initiation and sleep maintenance insomnia dating back to his university days. Initially his insomnia was intermittent, but with time it became a consistent feature of his sleep, though the severity varied. Over the years he had been given numerous short courses of hypnotics and, while they had worked well, his insomnia returned as soon as he had finished the course.

He managed to function well at work despite his fatigue, though his personal life suffered, as he was often too tired to socialize after work and spent much of the weekend lying in bed trying to catch up on lost sleep (with very little success). Seven years ago he moved to the United States and found the stress of living in a foreign country and the different working conditions very difficult. He was therefore no longer able to function on so little sleep and sought medical help. He was prescribed zolpidem 10 mg which he found very effective. He initially only took it on work nights, but as his job became busier and he started having to work weekends, he started taking it nightly.

Six months ago he returned to the United Kingdom. He registered with a GP and approached him for repeat prescriptions for the zolpidem. The GP was reluctant to prescribe the zolpidem for nightly use on a long-term basis and asked Mr S to try stopping it. Mr S explained that he had been taking the zolpidem for six years and had been using it nightly for the last four years. On one occasion he had forgotten to pack it when he went away for a holiday and hardly slept at all for two nights before he was able to obtain a prescription from a local doctor. He has tried sleeping the odd night here and there without the medication but has always had an awful night and gone back to taking the medication the following night.

Questions

1 Why did he have such a poor night's sleep each time he stopped the medication?

2 Was Mr S addicted to hypnotics?

3 What are the warning signs of hypnotic addiction or misuse?

4 How would you treat Mr S?

Answers

1. Why did he have such a poor night's sleep each time he stopped the medication?

The most obvious answer is that he still had an underlying insomnia. But it is more complex than that. He was probably also experiencing an element of rebound insomnia. Rebound insomnia is commonly seen when patients first stop or reduce their hypnotic. Their insomnia gets worse than it would have been had they never taken the hypnotic. Usually this rebound insomnia will recover after a few nights and the insomnia will return to its baseline level. However, many patients are unable to tolerate the wait and go back on to the hypnotic before the rebound insomnia has a chance to improve. They therefore compare their sleep on the hypnotic to their sleep during the rebound insomnia, rather than with their baseline insomnia. This reinforces the idea that they cannot sleep without the hypnotic. It is therefore essential that patients are informed about rebound insomnia when they start on hypnotics and are made aware that it is temporary.

Mr S did notice that his insomnia became significantly worse each time he reduced the dose of the medication and that it improved to some extent after a few nights. However, his sleep was never as good as it was on the medication and the cumulative fatigue made him increasingly anxious, which further affected his sleep.

The GP became extremely concerned that he had become addicted to the medication and referred Mr S to a substance misuse service to be 'detoxed'.

The substance misuse service put Mr S on a gradual reduction programme with weekly counselling. He successfully managed to stop the hypnotic over a period of eight weeks, but his insomnia became unbearable and he returned to the GP to ask for the prescription to be reinstated. He was unable to function at work and his job was at risk. The GP reluctantly agreed to reinstate the medication on a temporary basis and referred Mr S to the sleep service for a specialist opinion.

2. Was Mr S addicted to hypnotics?

This is an extremely difficult question to answer. Hypnotics do have the potential to become addictive and addiction to hypnotics is well documented in the literature. However, insomnia is often a long-term condition and once it has become chronic tends not to remit on its own. Therefore, when a patient stops the hypnotic it is to be expected that his insomnia will return and they are therefore likely to request further medication from their doctor. It may therefore be that Mr S was simply seeking the appropriate medication to treat his condition.

3. What are the warning signs of hypnotic addiction or misuse?

It is important to note that, as explained, continued use because the patient gets insomnia every time they stop is probably not sufficient to qualify them as misusing, or being dependent on, the drug. However, if the patient decides that they do want to stop the medication and are unable to do so, then clearly their relationship with the medication has become problematic. One of the hallmarks of addiction is continued use despite the drug causing more harm than good. Once again, it is important to differentiate between actual harm from the drug, such as severe side effects, and the doctor's anxiety about prescribing the drug.

Tolerance is always a worrying sign. Patients who find they need to escalate their dose in order to get the same effect are at increased risk of becoming dependent on the medication. One should also be on the lookout for patients who use multiple substances to induce or maintain sleep. Patients may combine prescription hypnotics with alcohol, over-the-counter antihistamines, antidepressants or anxiolytics. This is an extremely dangerous situation and significantly raises the risk of a fatal overdose as well as other adverse outcomes such as falls and car accidents. When patients buy hypnotics on the street or over the Internet this should be addressed as a matter of urgency. The quality and safety of these tablets is always a concern and of course there is no medical monitoring or supervision of their use.

Furthermore, one should always be on the lookout for patients who use hypnotics for reasons other than sleep, such as anxiety, or who engage in recreational use.

4. How would you treat Mr S?

The first issue to address is whether he needs to be treated. Many patients use hypnotics nightly for years without having any difficulties. However, it is always preferable to use non-medical interventions where possible. Some patients are able to stop hypnotics without medical assistance and some may even find that they sleep as well without medication as they did with it. However, patients are more likely to be successful if they engage in a supervised, gradual withdrawal programme. But withdrawing the medication successfully does not mean the insomnia is well controlled. When withdrawing one treatment, even one that is only partially effective, it makes sense that one should replace it with another effective treatment.

Mr S was therefore enrolled in a cognitive behaviour therapy for insomnia (CBT-I) programme. This was a six-week group programme where all the patients were long-term hypnotic users looking to reduce their medication. Studies comparing different reduction regimens for hypnotics are unfortunately lacking. It is therefore not possible to give firm recommendations about how fast one should reduce the medication, whether one should do the reduction before, during or after the CBT-I course, or whether it is better to reduce the medication by gradually reducing the dose or the frequency. In practice, we present all the possibilities to the patients and negotiate a programme that they feel will be realistic and will suit them best. What studies do exist generally use a reduction of 25% of the original dose every one to two weeks, and we use this as a starting point. We set targets and encourage the patient to reduce their medication by a certain amount each fortnight. However, these targets are flexible and sometimes patients will progress more quickly while at other times they may remain on a dose for a bit longer.

Most patients choose to do the dose reduction during the CBT-I course, as this allows them to get weekly supervision and support.

Mr S chose to do this and set a target of reducing by 25% every two weeks. We therefore changed his zolpidem from one 10 mg tablet to two 5 mg tablets. He was therefore able to reduce his dose by 25% by taking one and a half tablets, then one tablet and finally half a tablet. He did experience rebound insomnia after the first dose reduction, but as he now knew about rebound insomnia, and knew it was likely to resolve, he was able to persist with the reduction. The rebound insomnia improved after four nights, though his sleep was not quite as good as it had been on the full dose. However, as he started putting the CBT-I techniques into practice his sleep improved, which gave him the confidence to reduce the dose further.

By the end of the CBT-I course he had reduced his medication to 2.5 mg and was sleeping well. We explained that at such a low dose it was unlikely to be having a significant physiological effect and that any perceived benefit was likely to be largely down to a placebo effect. We advised that he start reducing the frequency of the medication and that he make a point of not taking it the night before big meetings or busy days to test his ability to sleep under pressure. However, at this point Mr S was feeling so confident that he decided to stop the medication altogether. He reported having two nights of worse sleep, which he attributed to the anxiety of not taking the medication, but then his sleep settled and at three month follow-up he was still sleeping well without any medication.

Learning points

Long-term hypnotic use and an inability to sleep well without hypnotics do not necessarily indicate addiction to the hypnotics. Insomnia is often a chronic disorder that requires long-term treatment.

However, tolerance, dose escalation, mixing medications or hypnotics with alcohol, or using the hypnotic during the day are warning signs of dependence.

If patients want to decrease their hypnotic use the best results are probably achieved through a gradual, supervised withdrawal in combination with CBT-I. If one is withdrawing a treatment, even a partially effective one, one should put another treatment in its place.

Rebound insomnia is a common consequence of reducing or stopping a hypnotic. This worsening of the insomnia is often very unpleasant and anxiety provoking, but it is almost always temporary. If the patient is forewarned about the rebound insomnia they are more likely to be able to endure it until their sleep recovers.

Further reading

Bélanger L, Belleville G, Morin C. Management of hypnotic discontinuation in chronic insomnia. Sleep Medicine Clinics 2009 Dec;4(4):583–92.

Hall-Porter JM, Curry DT, Walsh JK. Pharmacologic treatment of primary insomnia. Sleep Medicine Clinics 2010 Dec;5(4):609–25.

Riemann D, Perlis ML. The treatments of chronic insomnia: a review of benzodiazepine receptor agonists and psychological and behavioral therapies. Sleep Medicine Reviews 2009 Jun;13(3):205–14.

Case 55
My body clock cannot keep up

Mr V is a 36-year-old news editor who works for a 24-hour news TV station. He was referred to the sleep clinic by his employer's occupational health department after he started falling asleep at work. He worked a shift pattern that involved one of three shifts: 8.00 a.m. to 4.00 p.m. (early shift), 2.00 p.m. to 10.00 p.m. (late shift) and 9.00 p.m. to 9.00 a.m. (night shift). He had been working in his post for seven years and initially had performed very well, rapidly advancing to a more senior position. However, approximately a year before his presentation he started to have difficulty concentrating during night shifts. He made a number of uncharacteristic mistakes which led his managers to express their concern about his performance and it was agreed that they would monitor his work more closely. It was during this monitoring period that he was found asleep at his desk on three separate occasions. Mr V admitted that he was finding night shifts increasingly difficult, primarily because he was unable to sleep during the day between shifts. This had never been a problem before, but he was now struggling to get adequate sleep, which left him feeling fatigued and sleepy at night.

He was referred to occupational health who initially wondered if he was depressed, but a psychiatric consult found no evidence of a mood disorder, though they commented that he had an anxious disposition. The matter escalated when he started to have difficulty sleeping at night as well, leading to daytime fatigue. When he was found asleep at his desk twice during day shifts he was advised to take a month's leave and 'sort himself out'. Mr V decided the stress of his job was getting to him and so went to visit his parents in France for the month. He noticed that his sleep improved fairly quickly and he was able to sleep well at night and feel alert during the day. On returning to work he went on to day shifts for two weeks and his sleep remained good. He was therefore confident that the problem had been resolved. However, when he rotated on to night shifts he had trouble sleeping during the day again and, even when he rotated back to day shifts, his sleep remained poor. Within a month he was falling asleep at work again and was suspended from his job.

Questions

1 What is the likely diagnosis?
2 Can you design shift patterns to minimize the risk of shift work disorder (SWD)?
3 How would you treat Mr V's SWD?

Answers

1. What is the likely diagnosis?

SWD, a disorder which may affect over one-fifth of night workers and workers on rotating shifts. This is a circadian rhythm disorder leading to insomnia and/or excessive sleepiness, particularly during work shifts, leading to occupational or other dysfunction.

Humans have an internal circadian clock which is one of the major determinants of when we feel awake and when we feel sleepy. As diurnal creatures we are naturally predisposed to sleep at night and be awake during the day. This obviously makes it difficult to work nights, and most night workers will report periods of intense sleepiness and fatigue during night shifts that do not occur during the day. In addition to the difficulty of working at a time when the body expects to be asleep, it is also difficult to sleep at a time when the body expects to be awake. Therefore, despite being tired from a night shift (which is often longer than the day shift, as was the case for Mr V, and most doctors), the person may find it very difficult to go to sleep when they get home from work. Another complication is that when the worker is going home they may be exposed to bright morning light, which may have an alerting effect on the person and potentially confuse the body clock further.

Finally, it is often more difficult to sleep during the day than during the night. There is usually more light and noise during the day, which is likely to disrupt their sleep. There are also social factors such as the fact that they may need to sacrifice some of their sleep time to make phone calls to companies that are only open during the day, go to the bank, fetch the kids from school, etc.

Night work presents enough difficulties of its own. But when the person works rotating shifts an additional layer of complexity is added. Not only does the person have to cope with working unsociable hours, but these hours keep changing, usually at a pace too fast for the body clock to keep up. As a result, they may also find that they are sleepy at work when working day shifts and have difficulty sleeping at night.

SWD is not only problematic for the patient, but can have serious consequences for society as a whole. For example, pilots, truck drivers, doctors and nurses, police, air traffic controllers, train drivers and taxi drivers are all at high risk of SWD. As their alertness is adversely affected by the SWD it is concerning that it is so rarely recognized.

2. Can you design shift patterns to minimize the risk of SWD?

There is some controversy about which shift patterns are least likely to induce SWD. If the person does only a few days on each shift they will struggle to settle into the new schedule and, as soon as they do, they will rotate to a different schedule. On the one hand, doing a month of earlies, a month of lates and a month of nights gives the person's circadian rhythm a sporting chance of catching up with the work schedule. However, a month of nights can be gruelling, particularly if their daytime sleep is disturbed by environmental stimuli, and has a significant impact on their social lives. Most jobs use fairly rapidly rotating shifts, spending a few days on each shift. There are three ways these shifts can be organized:

- Anti-clockwise rotation—the person works progressively earlier shifts, e.g. four days late, four days early, four days nights, four days off.
- Clockwise rotation—the person works progressively later shifts, e.g. four days early, four days late, four days nights, four days off.
- Random shifts where there is no clear pattern. This pattern is often found even when the rota uses one of the above patterns, as people swap shifts to meet social commitments.

As a rule, the clockwise rotation is the best shift pattern. As most people have an inherent circadian rhythm that is slightly longer than 24 hours, it is easier to delay your circadian rhythm to advance it. Therefore, it is easier to adjust to a progressive delay in the shift pattern. It also means that when you move from one shift to another you have a longer break between the shifts. For example, if Mr V moves clockwise from an early to a late shift, there is a 22-hour break between the end of the early shift and the start of the late shift. But if he moves from the late to the early shift there are only ten hours between shifts. This would give him less time to sleep between shifts, so he may start the early shifts sleep deprived!

3. How would you treat Mr V's SWD?

There are four approaches to treating SWD: improving sleep between shifts, improving alertness during shifts, shifting the circadian rhythm to match the shift and designing the shift pattern to minimize the risk of SWD.

Improving sleep between shifts: The first interventions to put in place are the common sense things such as ensuring their environment is conducive to sleep, especially when they are sleeping during the day. This will often require the cooperation of their family. They should avoid caffeine for approximately six hours prior to the desired time of sleep onset. If their sleep is adversely affected by anxiety, then using cognitive behaviour therapy can be helpful. Some patients benefit from using hypnotics to establish their new sleep pattern when they change shifts and particularly when they are trying to sleep during the day.

Improving alertness during shifts: Timed naps are particularly helpful here. Naps can be timed to occur just prior to the start of the shift, in quiet periods during the shift and during periods when the circadian rhythm strongly predisposes one to sleepiness, e.g. at around 5.00 a.m. It should be noted that, as some people have an element of sleep inertia on waking from sleep, they should not nap if they may need to respond to emergencies immediately on waking. Judicious use of caffeine can be surprisingly effective and it can be used prior to the time they habitually feel sleepy to prevent the sleepiness occurring. Another possibility is to get exposure to bright light during the shift, as light has an alerting effect, and some patients find physical exercise to be helpful as well. In some cases stimulant medications such as modafinil are warranted and their use is supported by trial data.

Shifting the circadian rhythm to match the shift: This is often quite difficult, particularly in rapidly rotating shifts. As a rule of thumb, melatonin is given a few hours prior to the desired sleep period (though it should not be taken before driving home, as it is mildly sedative). Light exposure is timed to occur when the person first wakes up and they avoid light prior to going to bed (if necessary using dark glasses or welder's glasses).

Mr V had already taken the common sense steps of ensuring his sleep environment was dark and quiet, and he unplugged his phone to ensure he was not disturbed while sleeping during the day. He tried using hypnotics to help him sleep between shifts, and while this improved his sleep it did not particularly improve his alertness, especially during night shifts. He was also anxious about using hypnotics in the long term. We noted that his shift pattern was fairly random and wrote to his employers asking them to consider putting Mr V on a clockwise rotating shift pattern. We also advised them to facilitate timed naps during work. They initially agreed to the clockwise rotating shift but this fell apart after a month, as it required significant changes to everyone else's shifts and they were not willing to do this. They were not willing to facilitate planned naps, but said that all workers had a 45-minute break in the middle of their shift for 'lunch' and Mr V could use the bed in the first aid room to nap then instead of eating.

We gave Mr V melatonin 2 mg to be taken immediately on getting home from his shift and a light box to use immediately on waking. Although his shifts were too chaotic for us to have any realistic hope of shifting his circadian rhythm quickly enough to match his work pattern, we felt it was worth trying. He found the melatonin did improve his sleep and the light box had an alerting effect, so he started each shift feeling more awake than he had before. Mr V also used caffeine prior to the start of each shift and then again an hour prior to the times he felt most sleepy.

These interventions helped to a certain extent but he was still struggling, so our next step was to prescribe modafinil to help him stay awake during the shifts. This was initially very effective and he was coping much better at work. Unfortunately, after a few months he started to develop headaches from the modafinil and had to stop it. He was not keen on trying any other stimulants and had decided that he needed to change his lifestyle to fit his body clock, rather than the other way around. Therefore, with our support, he asked his employers to take him off night shifts permanently. They were not willing to do this unless he took a demotion and a significant cut in his salary.

After much soul-searching he decided his health was more important than the job and, with the help of his union, negotiated a severance package which he used to set himself up as a freelancer. He set himself very regular working hours and both his symptoms resolved completely. He was therefore discharged from the clinic.

Learning points

Shift work creates some unique problems for a person's sleep–wake cycle. Some people cope with this well, but many will develop SWD.

Designing shift patterns to better match the workers' circadian rhythms is a sensible intervention. In practice this means rotating the shifts clockwise, i.e. rotating to later shifts rather than earlier shifts.

Interventions involve improving sleep between shifts, improving alertness during shifts and shifting the circadian rhythm to better match the shift pattern.

Some patients will not improve despite the above interventions and therefore there are circumstances where the best treatment is to stop doing shift work.

Further reading

Crowley SJ et al. Complete or partial circadian re-entrainment improves performance, alertness, and mood during night-shift work. Sleep 2004 Sep;27(6):1077–87.

Owens JA, Veasey SC, Rosen RC. Physician, heal thyself: sleep, fatigue, and medical education. Sleep 2001 Aug;24(5):493–5.

Wright KP, Bogan RK, Wyatt JK. Shift work and the assessment and management of shift work disorder (SWD). Sleep Med Rev 2013 Feb;17(1):41–54.

List of cases by diagnosis

Section 1: Snoring and sleep-disordered breathing

1. Snoring and witnessed apnoea in a 70-year-old thin man
2. An obese post-menopausal woman snored like a tank
3. Severe OSA in an overweight Chinese man—craniofacial features
4. Unable to throw a cricket ball and could not breathe at night
5. A sleepy bus driver
6. Rapid onset daytime sleep presenting as transient loss of consciousness
7. Unexplained breathlessness and pulmonary arterial hypertension in an obese man
8. Post-operative apnoeas and hypoxia due to undiagnosed OSA
9. Polycythemia got better with CPAP
10. Hyperphagia and sleep disorder in Prader–Willi Syndrome
11. Shot in the head—acquired hypothalamic syndrome
12. Collapsed in a café: acute respiratory failure
13. Overlap syndrome—COPD and OSA
14. Neuropsychological impairment in a psychoanalyst with post-polio syndrome
15. Nocturnal choking in a patient with a goitre and retrosternal extension
16. OSA persists despite removal of a pituitary tumour causing acromegaly
17. CPAP transformed my life
18. Persistent daytime sleepiness despite CPAP
19. CPAP intolerance and non-compliance treatment with MAS
20. Will not use CPAP—ends up with tracheostomy
21. Bariatric surgery cures sleep apnoea
22. Sleep disturbance and daytime sleepiness persists in a snorer despite CPAP—PLMS
23. Worrying pauses in breath without choking and snoring—CSA
24. Irresistible daytime sleepiness in a young obese woman

Section 2: Snoring and OSA: role of dental and ENT surgeons

25. Contribution of facial skeletal pattern to sleep apnoea

26. MAS therapy for severe OSAHS

27. Effectiveness, compliance and side effects of MAS therapy

28. Allergic rhinitis

29. Nasal polyposis

30. Septoplasty

31. UARS

32. Laser Assisted Uvulopalatoplasty (LAUP)/tonsillectomy

33. Epiglottic trapdoor

34. Tracheostomy

Section 3: Neurological sleep disorders

35. Sleep groaning

36. Nocturnal punch and fight

37. Jumpy legs

38. Episodic weak legs in a sleepy man

39. Just sleepy all the time

40. Moving and thrashing around during sleep

41. Panic attacks during sleep

42. Frozen in sleep

43. Confused, irritable and sleepy young man

44. Chattering teeth during sleep

45. Sexsomnia

Section 4: Insomnia and circadian rhythm disorders

46. I keep falling asleep at family dinners

47. I have not slept in years

48. Spending too long in bed

49. A sleep cycle that keeps moving

50. My body is in London but my body clock is in New York

51. A very, very long day

52. Sleep and alcohol abuse

53. Choosing and using hypnotics

54. Please see this patient who is addicted to sleeping pills

55. My body clock cannot keep up

List of cases by principal clinical features at diagnosis

List of cases by aetiological mechanisms

Index

Notes

vs. indicates a comparison or differential diagnosis

Page numbers suffixed with 't' refer to details in table, 'f' in figures.

A

abdominal movement, OSA diagnosis 12

abdominal wall muscles, post-polio syndrome 98

acetazolamide, CSA treatment 155, 156

acoustic rhinometry, rhinitis 198

acquired hypothalamic syndrome
  case study 73–80
  clinical features 79
  CPAP 73
  definition 79
  EDS 73–74
  nocturnal hypoxia 73
  obesity 73–74

acromegaly
  case study 107–110
  craniofacial abnormalities 108
  growth hormone 108
  insulin-like growth factor 108
  MRI 109f
  OSA 108
  treatment 108
  see also pituitary tumours

actigraphy
  ASPS diagnosis 272
  DSPS investigations 309
  non-24-hour sleep–wake syndrome 301–302, 301f

acute hypercapnic respiratory failure (AHRF)
  case study 81–87
  causes 85, 85t
  chest X-ray 81, 82f
  clinical features 84, 84t
  C-reactive protein (CRP) 81
  CT 81
  Glasgow Coma Scale (GCS) 81
  OSA risk from 86–87
  sleep study 81–82, 83f
  white cell count 81

adaptive servo-ventilation (ASV), CSA treatment 156

advanced sleep phase syndrome (ASPS)
  case study 271–276
  diagnosis 272–273
  treatment 273

aero-allergens 188

age, OSA 8

AHI *see* apnoea hypopnea index (AHI)

AHRF *see* acute hypercapnic respiratory failure (AHRF)

airflow obstruction 53

alcohol abuse
  case study 321–328
  detoxification 322
  effects on sleep 324
  history 321–322
  OSA 103, 105–106
  treatment 324–326
  see also alcohol-induced hypotonia

alcohol-induced hypotonia 105–106
  oximetry 106f

allergen avoidance, allergic rhinitis 188–189

allergen-specific IgE blood tests 188

allergic rhinitis 129
  allergen avoidance 188–189
  case study 185–190
  investigations 187–188
  pharmacological treatment 189–190
  skin prick testing 187, 187f

ALS (amyotrophic lateral sclerosis), OSA 30

alternative remedies 329

American Academy of Sleep Medicine, sleep assessment 36

amphetamines, narcolepsy treatment 242

amyotrophic lateral sclerosis (ALS), OSA 30